# KATE HALE

## Minimalist Home

*Transforming Your Living Space into a Haven of Simplicity*

Copyright © 2024 by KATE HALE

All rights reserved. No part of this publication may be reproduced, stored or transmitted in any form or by any means, electronic, mechanical, photocopying, recording, scanning, or otherwise without written permission from the publisher. It is illegal to copy this book, post it to a website, or distribute it by any other means without permission.

First edition

This book was professionally typeset on Reedsy.
Find out more at reedsy.com

# Contents

# Introduction

I n recent years, the concept of minimalism has taken the world by storm, captivating people from all walks of life with its promise of a simpler, more purposeful existence. At its core, minimalism is about living with intention, focusing on what truly matters, and letting go of the excess that clutters our lives. While minimalism can be applied to various aspects of life, one of the most impact ways to embrace this philosophy is by transforming your living space into a minimalist haven.

The rise of minimalism can be attributed to several factors. In our fast-paced, consumer-driven society, many people have found themselves overwhelmed by the sheer volume of possessions they have accumulated over the years. The constant pressure to buy more, upgrade to the latest trends, and keep up with the Joneses has left us feeling stressed, unfulfilled, and disconnected from what truly matters. Minimalism offers a way out of this cycle, inviting us to reassess our priorities and focus on the things that bring us genuine joy and fulfillment.

One of the most compelling reasons to embrace minimalism in your home is the myriad of benefits it offers. A minimalist living space can have a profound impact on your physical, mental, and emotional well-being. When you declutter your home and keep only the items that serve a purpose or spark joy, you create a sense of clarity and calm that permeates every aspect of your life.

A minimalist home is easier to clean and maintain, saving you time and energy that can be better spent on the things you love. With fewer possessions to manage, you'll find yourself less stressed and more focused on the present moment. A clutter-free environment also promotes better sleep, as a tidy bedroom creates a peaceful atmosphere conducive to relaxation and rest.

Moreover, embracing minimalism in your home can lead to significant financial benefits. By consuming less and being more intentional with your purchases, you can save money and reduce debt. Instead of constantly buying new items to fill your space, you can invest in experiences, relationships, and personal growth, cultivating a richer and more fulfilling life.

Beyond the personal benefits, minimalism also has positive implications for the environment. By reducing consumption and waste, you can lessen your ecological footprint and contribute to a more sustainable future. Minimalism encourages us to be mindful of our impact on the planet and to make choices that prioritize long-term value over short-term gratification.

This book is for anyone who yearns for a simpler, more intentional way of living. Whether you're a busy professional looking to create a peaceful retreat from the chaos of daily life, a family seeking to foster a more connected and harmonious home, or a retiree ready to downsize and embrace a new chapter, the principles and strategies outlined in this book will guide you on your journey toward a minimalist home.

Throughout the pages of this book, you'll learn how to cultivate a minimalist mindset, letting go of the beliefs and habits that have been holding you back from living your best life. You'll discover practical decluttering techniques and strategies for every room in your home, making the process of simplifying your space manageable and achievable.

But minimalism is about more than just getting rid of stuff. It's about being intentional with what you choose to keep and how you design your living space. This book will introduce you to the principles of minimalist design, helping you create a home that is not only functional and organized but also beautiful and reflective of your personal style.

As you progress through your minimalist home transformation, you'll learn how to maintain a clutter-free space and adopt habits that support a minimalist lifestyle. You'll explore the benefits of living minimally, from increased time and financial freedom to reduced stress and improved well-being.

By the end of this book, you'll have the tools, knowledge, and inspiration to transform your living space into a haven of simplicity and purpose. You'll be well on your way to experiencing the joy and fulfillment that comes from living with less and focusing on what truly matters.

It's important to remember that minimalism is a personal journey, and there is no one-size-fits-all approach. The strategies and ideas presented in this book are meant to be adapted to your unique circumstances and goals. Whether you choose to embrace minimalism fully or simply incorporate some of its principles into your life, any step toward simplifying your home is a step in the right direction.

As you embark on this trans formative journey, be patient with yourself and celebrate the small victories along the way. Decluttering and simplifying your home is not an overnight process, but rather a gradual shift toward a more intentional and meaningful way of living.

Throughout this book, you'll find practical tips, real-life examples, and inspirational stories to keep you motivated and on track. You'll also discover a supportive community of like-minded individuals who are on their own minimalist journeys, reminding you that you are not alone in your pursuit of a simpler, more fulfilling life.

So, whether you're a minimalist novice or a seasoned simplifies, this book is your guide to creating a home that reflects your values, supports your goals, and brings you lasting joy and contentment. By embracing minimalism in your living space, you're not just transforming your home; you're transforming your life.

Get ready to let go of the excess, focus on what truly matters, and experience the freedom and happiness that comes from living with less. Your minimalist home awaits!

# The Minimalist Mindset

Before diving into the practical aspects of transforming your living space, it's essential to understand the foundation upon which a minimalist home is built: the minimalist mindset. In this section, we'll explore the definition and principles of minimalism, dispel common misconceptions, and examine minimalism as a lifestyle choice. By cultivating a minimalist mindset, you'll be better equipped to navigate the challenges and reap the benefits of creating a minimalist home.

Understanding Minimalism

Definition and Principles of Minimalism

At its core, minimalism is a philosophy that encourages individuals to live with intention, focusing on what truly matters and letting go of the excess that clutters their lives. It's about prioritizing experiences, relationships, and personal growth over material possessions and societal expectations.

The principles of minimalism can be distilled into three key ideas:

1. Intersectionality: Minimalists make deliberate choices about what they allow into their lives, ensuring that each item, commitment, and relationship serves a purpose and aligns with their values.

2. Simplicity: By stripping away the unnecessary, minimalists create space

for what truly matters. They seek to simplify their lives in all aspects, from their possessions to their schedules and relationships.

3. Contentment: Minimalists find joy and fulfillment in living with less, recognizing that happiness comes from within and is not dependent on external factors or material possessions.

These principles can be applied to various aspects of life, from personal finance and career choices to relationships and, of course, one's living space.

Misconceptions about Minimalism

Despite its growing popularity, minimalism is often misunderstood. Let's address some common misconceptions about minimalism:

1. Minimalism is about deprivation: One of the most pervasive myths about minimalism is that it's about depriving oneself of joy and comfort. In reality, minimalism is about letting go of what doesn't serve you to make room for what does. It's about living with intention and finding fulfillment in experiences and relationships rather than material possessions.

2. Minimalists live in stark, empty spaces: While some minimalists prefer a highly streamlined aesthetic, minimalism is not synonymous with a particular style. A minimalist home can be warm, inviting, and reflective of one's personal taste. The focus is on keeping only what is essential and meaningful, not on achieving a certain "look."

3. Minimalism is only for single people or those without children: Minimalism can be adapted to suit any lifestyle, including families with children. In fact, many families find that embracing minimalism helps create a more peaceful, organized, and connected home environment.

4. Minimalism is a one-time event: Minimalism is not a destination but

rather an ongoing journey. It requires a shift in mindset and a commitment to living intentionally. While decluttering is an essential part of the process, minimalism is a lifestyle that extends beyond the initial purge.

By understanding these misconceptions and the true essence of minimalism, you can approach your minimalist home transformation with a clear and open mind.

Minimalism as a Lifestyle Choice

Embracing minimalism is a personal choice that reflects one's values, priorities, and aspirations. It's a lifestyle that extends beyond the confines of one's living space and permeates all aspects of life.

When you choose minimalism as a lifestyle, you are making a conscious decision to:

1. Live with intention: Minimalism encourages you to be deliberate in your choices, aligning your actions with your values and goals. This intersectionality applies to your possessions, relationships, commitments, and use of time.

2. Prioritize experiences over things: Minimalists recognize that lasting happiness and fulfillment come from meaningful experiences, personal growth, and deep connections with others. They prioritize investing in experiences and relationships rather than accumulating material possessions.

3. Cultivate gratitude and contentment: By letting go of the excess and focusing on what truly matters, minimalists develop a deep sense of gratitude for what they have. They find contentment in the present moment, rather than constantly seeking happiness in the next purchase or milestone.

4. Embrace simplicity: Minimalism invites you to simplify your life in all

areas, from your daily routines and commitments to your financial habits and environmental impact. By streamlining your life, you create space for what truly brings you joy and fulfillment.

5. Live sustainably: Minimalism and sustainability go hand in hand. By consuming less, minimalists reduce their ecological footprint and contribute to a more sustainable future. They prioritize quality over quantity, choosing items that are durable, versatile, and ethically produced.

Embracing minimalism as a lifestyle choice requires a shift in perspective and a willingness to let go of societal expectations and pressures. It's a personal journey that looks different for everyone, but the core principles of intersectionality, simplicity, and contentment remain the same.

As you embark on your minimalist home transformation, remember that the process extends beyond decluttering your physical space. It's an opportunity to reassess your priorities, cultivate a mindset of abundance, and align your living environment with your values and goals.

In the following chapters, we'll explore practical strategies for decluttering, designing, and maintaining a minimalist home. But remember, the foundation of a truly minimalist home lies in the mindset you bring to the process. By embracing the principles of minimalism and making intentional choices, you'll not only transform your living space but also create a more meaningful and fulfilling life.

So, let's dive in and explore the trans formative power of a minimalist mindset in creating a home that reflects your true priorities and brings you lasting joy and contentment.

# Discovering Your "Why"

Before embarking on your minimalist home transformation, it's crucial to take a step back and reflect on your motivations and goals. Understanding your "why" will serve as a guiding light throughout your journey, helping you stay focused and committed when challenges arise. In this section, we'll explore how to identify your values and priorities, set intentions for your minimalist journey, and visualize your ideal living space.

Identifying Your Values and Priorities

Your values and priorities are the foundation upon which your minimalist lifestyle will be built. They serve as a compass, guiding you towards what truly matters and helping you make intentional choices about what to keep and what to let go of in your home and life.

To identify your values and priorities, start by asking yourself the following questions:

1. What matters most to you in life? Consider the relationships, experiences, and personal qualities that bring you the greatest sense of fulfillment and joy.

2. What do you want more of in your life? Reflect on the aspects of your life that you wish to cultivate and grow, such as time with loved ones, personal growth, or creative pursuits.

3. What do you want less of in your life? Think about the things that drain your energy, cause stress, or distract you from what truly matters, such as clutter, over scheduling, or negative relationships.

4. What legacy do you want to leave? Consider how you want to be remembered and the impact you wish to have on others and the world around you.

As you reflect on these questions, make a list of the values and priorities that emerge. Some examples might include:

- Family and relationships
    - Health and well-being
    - Personal growth and learning
    - Creativity and self-expression
    - Environmental sustainability
    - Financial stability and freedom
    - Meaningful work and contribution

Once you have identified your core values and priorities, rank them in order of importance. This exercise will help you gain clarity on what truly matters to you and serve as a guide for your minimalist home transformation.

Setting Intentions for Your Minimalist Journey

With your values and priorities in mind, it's time to set intentions for your minimalist journey. Intentions are different from goals in that they focus on the present moment and the overall direction you want to move in, rather than a specific endpoint.

When setting intentions, consider the following:

1. What do you hope to gain from embracing minimalism? Think about the

benefits you seek, such as more time, space, freedom, or peace of mind.

2. How do you want to feel in your minimalist home? Consider the emotions and sensations you wish to cultivate, such as calm, comfort, inspiration, or connection.

3. What habits and practices do you want to embrace? Reflect on the daily routines and rituals that will support your minimalist lifestyle, such as decluttering regularly, practicing gratitude, or simplifying your schedule.

Some examples of intentions for your minimalist journey might include:

- "I intend to create a home that feels peaceful, spacious, and reflective of my true priorities."
  - "I intend to let go of the excess in my life, both physically and emotionally, to make room for what truly matters."
  - "I intend to cultivate a deeper sense of gratitude and contentment with what I have."
  - "I intend to simplify my life so that I have more time and energy for the people and pursuits that bring me joy."

Write down your intentions and place them somewhere you'll see them regularly, such as on your bathroom mirror or refrigerator. Use them as a reminder of your "why" and a source of motivation throughout your minimalist home transformation.

Visualizing Your Ideal Living Space

Now that you have identified your values and priorities and set intentions for your minimalist journey, it's time to bring your vision to life by visualizing your ideal living space.

Visualization is a powerful tool for manifesting your desires and staying motivated throughout the decluttering and design process. By creating a clear mental picture of your minimalist home, you'll have a tangible goal to work towards and a source of inspiration when challenges arise.

To visualize your ideal living space, find a quiet, comfortable place where you won't be disturbed. Close your eyes and take a few deep breaths, allowing yourself to relax and let go of any distractions or worries.

Now, imagine yourself walking through the front door of your minimalist home. What do you see, hear, feel, and smell? Consider the following aspects of your ideal living space:

1. Layout and flow: Visualize the overall layout of your home, including the placement of furniture and the flow between rooms. Consider how the space feels open, airy, and uncluttered.

2. Color palette and lighting: Imagine the colors and textures that create a sense of calm and harmony in your home. Consider how natural light fills the space and how cozy, warm lighting creates a welcoming atmosphere in the evening.

3. Furnishings and decor: Picture the essential pieces of furniture that serve a purpose and bring you joy. Visualize the carefully curated decor that reflects your personal style and values, such as meaningful artwork, cherished photos, or natural elements.

4. Organization and storage: Imagine how each item in your home has a designated place and how easy it is to find what you need. Consider the clever storage solutions that keep your space clutter-free and functional.

5. Atmosphere and ambiance: Envision the overall feeling of your minimalist home, such as the sense of peace, comfort, and contentment that permeates the space. Consider how your home supports your daily routines and rituals,

such as a cozy reading nook or a serene meditation corner.

As you visualize your ideal living space, engage all of your senses and make the experience as vivid and detailed as possible. Notice how you feel in this space – the sense of ease, clarity, and joy that comes from living in a home that reflects your true priorities.

After you've spent some time visualizing your minimalist home, open your eyes and take a few moments to journal about your experience. Write down the key elements that stood out to you, the emotions you felt, and any insights or inspirations that arose.

Use this visualization as a touchstone throughout your minimalist home transformation, returning to it whenever you need a reminder of your "why" or a boost of motivation. Remember, your ideal living space is not a static endpoint but rather an evolving reflection of your values, priorities, and intentions.

By discovering your "why," setting intentions, and visualizing your ideal living space, you lay the foundation for a successful and fulfilling minimalist home transformation. With a clear sense of purpose and a compelling vision to guide you, you'll be well-equipped to navigate the challenges and embrace the joys of creating a home that reflects your authentic self.

In the next section, we'll explore the common obstacles that can arise during the minimalist journey and strategies for overcoming them with grace and resilience. Remember, transformation is a process, and every step you take towards your ideal living space is a victory to be celebrated.

# Overcoming Obstacles and Embracing Change

As you embark on your minimalist home transformation, it's essential to recognize that change, even positive change, can be challenging. Along the way, you may encounter obstacles that test your resolve and make you question your commitment to minimalism. In this section, we'll explore common challenges and how to overcome them, strategies for dealing with sentimental attachments, and the importance of involving family members in the process.

Common Challenges and How to Overcome Them

Transforming your living space and adopting a minimalist lifestyle is a significant undertaking that requires patience, perseverance, and a willingness to step outside your comfort zone. Let's explore some of the common challenges you may face and strategies for overcoming them:

1. Overwhelm and decision fatigue: The process of decluttering and simplifying your home can be overwhelming, especially if you have a lot of possessions or have been accumulating clutter for years. You may find yourself feeling paralyzed by the sheer number of decisions you need to make about what to keep and what to let go of.

To overcome this challenge, break the process down into small, manageable steps. Focus on one room, one category of items, or even one drawer at a time. Set a timer for decluttering sessions and take breaks when needed. Celebrate your progress, no matter how small, and remind yourself that each item you let go of brings you one step closer to your ideal living space.

2. Fear of letting go: Letting go of possessions can be emotionally challenging, even when those items no longer serve a purpose or bring you joy. You may fear that letting go of certain items means letting go of memories, security, or a part of your identity.

To overcome this fear, practice self-compassion and acknowledge that these feelings are normal and valid. Remind yourself that your memories and experiences are not tied to physical objects and that letting go of possessions does not diminish their significance. Focus on the benefits of letting go, such as creating space for what truly matters and cultivating a sense of lightness and freedom.

3. Resistance to change: Change can be uncomfortable, even when it's self-initiated. As you transform your living space and embrace a minimalist lifestyle, you may find yourself resisting the process, questioning your decisions, or slipping back into old habits.

To overcome resistance, remind yourself of your "why" and the intentions you set for your minimalist journey. Surround yourself with supportive resources, such as books, podcasts, or online communities, that inspire and motivate you. Practice self-compassion and recognize that setbacks are a natural part of the process. Celebrate your successes, no matter how small, and focus on the progress you've made rather than the challenges you face.

4. External pressures and expectations: As you embrace minimalism, you may encounter resistance or criticism from family members, friends, or society at large. Others may not understand your choices or may pressure you to conform to their expectations.

To overcome external pressures, set clear boundaries and communicate your values and intentions with kindness and confidence. Surround yourself with supportive individuals who respect your choices and cheer you on. Remember that your minimalist journey is a personal one and that you don't need to justify your decisions to others.

By anticipating these common challenges and developing strategies for overcoming them, you'll be better equipped to navigate the ups and downs of your minimalist home transformation with grace and resilience.

Dealing with Sentimental Attachments

One of the most significant obstacles to decluttering and embracing minimalism is dealing with sentimental attachments to possessions. These items, such as family heirlooms, childhood mementos, or gifts from loved ones, can hold deep emotional significance and be difficult to let go of, even when they no longer serve a practical purpose or align with your current values and lifestyle.

Here are some strategies for dealing with sentimental attachments:

1. Acknowledge the emotions: Allow yourself to feel the emotions that arise when considering letting go of a sentimental item. Acknowledge the memories and significance attached to the object and the difficulty of parting with it.

2. Reflect on the true source of the sentiment: Ask yourself whether the sentiment lies in the object itself or in the memories and experiences it represents. Recognize that your memories and the love of the person who gave you the item will remain even if you let go of the physical object.

3. Consider the item's current role in your life: Reflect on whether the sentimental item plays an active role in your life or whether it is simply

taking up space. Consider whether holding onto the item aligns with your current values and priorities.

4. Find alternative ways to honor the sentiment: If you decide to let go of a sentimental item, consider alternative ways to honor the memory or sentiment it represents. This might include taking a photo of the item, writing about the memory or person associated with it, or creating a small, curated display of truly cherished mementos.

5. Practice gratitude and letting go: As you let go of sentimental items, practice gratitude for the role they have played in your life and the memories they hold. Recognize that letting go creates space for new experiences and growth and that the sentiment and love remain even as the physical object is released.

Remember, dealing with sentimental attachments is a deeply personal process, and there is no right or wrong way to approach it. Be patient and compassionate with yourself, and trust that as you continue to clarify your values and priorities, you'll find a way to honor your sentimental attachments while still embracing the benefits of a minimalist lifestyle.

Involving Family Members in the Process

Transforming your living space into a minimalist home is a personal journey, but if you share your home with family members, it's essential to involve them in the process. When everyone in the household is on board and actively participating, the transition to minimalism can be smoother, more successful, and more sustainable in the long run.

Here are some strategies for involving family members in your minimalist home transformation:

1. Communicate your intentions and values: Have an open and honest

conversation with your family members about your desire to embrace minimalism and transform your living space. Share your motivations, values, and the benefits you believe minimalism will bring to your household.

2. Listen to their concerns and perspectives: Encourage your family members to share their thoughts, concerns, and perspectives on minimalism and the changes you're proposing. Listen with an open mind and a willingness to find common ground.

3. Find shared values and priorities: Identify the values and priorities that you and your family members share, such as more quality time together, less stress and chaos in the home, or a greater focus on experiences over possessions. Use these shared values as a foundation for your minimalist journey.

4. Start with communal spaces: Begin your minimalist home transformation with shared living spaces, such as the living room, kitchen, and family room. Work together to declutter and simplify these areas, involving everyone in the decision-making process and ensuring that each person's needs and preferences are considered.

5. Respect individual spaces and belongings: As you move into more personal spaces, such as bedrooms and offices, respect each family member's autonomy and attachment to their belongings. Encourage and support their individual minimalist journeys, but don't force or pressure them to let go of items they're not ready to release.

6. Make it fun and rewarding: Turn your minimalist home transformation into a fun and rewarding experience for the whole family. Create challenges or games around decluttering, celebrate milestones and successes, and plan enjoyable experiences or treats with the time and resources you save through minimalism.

7. Lead by example: As you embrace minimalism in your personal spaces and habits, lead by example and demonstrate the benefits of a minimalist lifestyle. Share your experiences, challenges, and triumphs with your family members and invite them to join you in creating a home and life that reflects your shared values and priorities.

Remember, involving family members in your minimalist home transformation is an ongoing process that requires patience, communication, and compromise. By approaching the journey with compassion, respect, and a willingness to adapt, you can create a minimalist home that supports the well-being and happiness of every member of your household.

Embracing change and overcoming obstacles is an integral part of the minimalist journey. By anticipating common challenges, developing strategies for dealing with sentimental attachments, and involving family members in the process, you'll be well-equipped to navigate the ups and downs of your minimalist home transformation with grace, resilience, and a sense of shared purpose.

As you continue to clarify your values, set intentions, and take action towards your ideal living space, remember that progress is more important than perfection. Celebrate your successes, learn from your setbacks, and trust that each step you take brings you closer to a home and life that reflects your authentic self and the things that matter most.

In the next section, we'll dive into the practical aspects of decluttering your home, exploring strategies and techniques for simplifying your living space and letting go of the excess that no longer serves you. Armed with a clear sense of purpose and a toolkit for overcoming obstacles, you'll be ready to take on the challenges and reap the rewards of your minimalist home transformation.

# The Art of Decluttering

Decluttering is a fundamental aspect of creating a minimalist home. It involves removing the excess, letting go of items that no longer serve you, and creating space for what truly matters. In this section, we'll explore the benefits of decluttering, the KonMari Method and other decluttering techniques, and how to create a decluttering plan that works for you.

Benefits of Decluttering

Decluttering your home offers numerous benefits that extend beyond the physical space. Here are some of the key advantages of removing the excess and simplifying your surroundings:

1. Reduced stress and anxiety: A cluttered environment can be overwhelming and contribute to feelings of stress and anxiety. By decluttering your home, you create a sense of order and calm that promotes relaxation and peace of mind.

2. Increased focus and productivity: When your living space is cluttered and disorganized, it can be challenging to focus on tasks and be productive. Decluttering eliminates distractions and creates an environment that supports concentration and efficiency.

3. Enhanced sense of control: Clutter can leave you feeling overwhelmed

and out of control. By decluttering, you take charge of your environment and make intentional choices about what you allow into your space, fostering a sense of empowerment and control.

4. Improved health and well-being: A cluttered home can harbor dust, allergens, and other irritants that can negatively impact your physical health. Decluttering promotes a cleaner, healthier living space that supports your overall well-being.

5. Greater appreciation for what you have: When you remove the excess and surround yourself only with items that truly matter, you develop a deeper appreciation for the things you choose to keep. Decluttering helps you cultivate gratitude and contentment with what you have.

6. Easier maintenance and cleaning: A minimalist home with fewer possessions is easier to maintain and clean, saving you time and energy in the long run. Decluttering streamlines your cleaning routine and allows you to focus on enjoying your living space rather than constantly tidying up.

7. Increased space and functionality: By removing the clutter, you free up physical space in your home, making it feel larger, more open, and more functional. Decluttering allows you to optimize your living space and make the most of the square footage you have.

8. Financial benefits: Decluttering can have financial benefits, such as reducing the urge to buy more stuff, uncovering forgotten items that can be repurposed or sold, and avoiding the costs associated with storing and maintaining excess possessions.

9. Environmental sustainability: By decluttering and consuming less, you reduce your environmental impact and contribute to a more sustainable future. Decluttering encourages you to make mindful choices about your possessions and consider the life cycle of the items you bring into your home.

10. Emotional and mental freedom: Letting go of physical clutter can also help you release emotional and mental baggage. Decluttering creates space for personal growth, self-reflection, and new experiences, promoting a sense of lightness and freedom.

By recognizing the numerous benefits of decluttering, you can approach the process with a sense of purpose and motivation, knowing that the effort you put into simplifying your home will pay off in countless ways.

The KonMari Method and Other Decluttering Techniques

When it comes to decluttering your home, there are various methods and techniques to choose from. One of the most popular and effective approaches is the KonMari Method, developed by Japanese organizing consultant Marie Kondo. Here's an overview of the KonMari Method and other decluttering techniques:

1. The KonMari Method:
   - Tidying by category: The KonMari Method involves decluttering by category (e.g., clothes, books, papers) rather than by room. This approach allows you to see the full extent of your possessions in each category and make more informed decisions about what to keep.
   - Sparking joy: The core principle of the KonMari Method is to keep only those items that "spark joy." When decluttering, you hold each item and ask yourself whether it brings you genuine happiness and fulfillment. If not, you thank the item for its service and let it go.
   - Folding and organizing: After decluttering, the KonMari Method emphasizes the importance of proper folding and storage techniques to maximize space and maintain a tidy, visually appealing home.

2. The Four Box Method:
   - Sort items into four categories: With the Four Box Method, you declutter by sorting your possessions into four categories: keep, donate, sell, and trash.

This approach helps you make quick, decisive choices about each item and ensures that everything has a designated destination.

- Tackle one room at a time: Unlike the KonMari Method, the Four Box Method involves decluttering room by room, allowing you to see progress and feel a sense of accomplishment as you complete each space.

3. The One-In-One-Out Rule:

- Maintain balance: The One-In-One-Out Rule is a simple but effective technique for maintaining a clutter-free home. For every new item you bring into your space, you commit to removing one item in the same category. This approach helps you be mindful of your consumption and prevents the accumulation of excess possessions over time.

4. The 90/90 Rule:

- Evaluate the relevance of items: The 90/90 Rule asks you to consider whether you have used an item in the past 90 days or whether you plan to use it in the next 90 days. If the answer to both questions is no, it's likely that the item is not essential to your life and can be let go.

5. The Minimalist Game:

- Make decluttering fun: Developed by The Minimalists, Joshua Fields Millburn and Ryan Nicodemus, the Minimalist Game turns decluttering into a 30-day challenge. On day one, you remove one item; on day two, two items; and so on. This approach gamifies the decluttering process and encourages you to build momentum as you progress through the month.

Remember, the most effective decluttering technique is the one that resonates with you and your unique needs and preferences. Experiment with different methods and adapt them to suit your lifestyle and goals. The key is to find a process that helps you make intentional choices about your possessions and create a living space that reflects your values and priorities.

Creating a Decluttering Plan

Decluttering your entire home can feel overwhelming, especially if you have a significant amount of possessions or have been accumulating clutter for years. Creating a decluttering plan breaks the process down into manageable steps and helps you stay focused and motivated throughout your minimalist home transformation. Here's how to create a decluttering plan that works for you:

1. Set your intentions and goals: Before diving into the decluttering process, take some time to clarify your intentions and goals. Consider what you hope to achieve through decluttering, such as creating a more peaceful living space, reducing stress, or simplifying your life. Write down your goals and refer to them often to stay motivated and on track.

2. Choose a decluttering method: Decide which decluttering method or combination of methods you want to use, such as the KonMari Method, the Four Box Method, or the Minimalist Game. Consider your personality, lifestyle, and the amount of time you have available to dedicate to decluttering.

3. Break the process down into manageable steps: Divide your decluttering plan into smaller, manageable steps to avoid feeling overwhelmed. You can break the process down by room, category, or time frame, depending on your chosen method. For example, you might plan to declutter your wardrobe in week one, your books in week two, and your kitchen in week three.

4. Create a timeline: Establish a realistic timeline for your decluttering plan, taking into account your daily commitments and the size of your home. Be specific about when you will start and finish each step of the process, and build in some flexibility for unexpected challenges or setbacks.

5. Gather necessary supplies: Before starting the decluttering process, gather the supplies you'll need, such as boxes or bags for sorting items, labels, and cleaning materials. Having everything you need on hand will help you stay focused and efficient.

6. Enlist support: Consider enlisting the support of family members, friends, or a professional organizer to help you stay accountable and motivated throughout the decluttering process. Having someone to share the experience with can make it more enjoyable and provide a fresh perspective when making decisions about your possessions.

7. Start with easy wins: Begin your decluttering plan with areas or categories that feel relatively easy to tackle, such as expired food in your pantry or clothes that no longer fit. These quick wins will build momentum and give you a sense of accomplishment early in the process.

8. Schedule regular decluttering sessions: Incorporate decluttering into your regular routine by scheduling specific times to work on your plan. Block out time on your calendar and treat these sessions as non-negotiable commitments to your minimalist home transformation.

9. Celebrate your progress: As you complete each step of your decluttering plan, take a moment to celebrate your progress and acknowledge the hard work you've put in. Recognizing your achievements, no matter how small, will help you stay motivated and focused on your end goal.

10. Reassess and adjust as needed: As you work through your decluttering plan, be open to reassessing and adjusting your approach as needed. If something isn't working or you encounter unexpected challenges, don't be afraid to modify your plan or seek additional support.

Remember, creating a decluttering plan is a personal process that should be tailored to your unique needs, preferences, and goals. Be patient with yourself and trust that each step you take brings you closer to the minimalist home you envision.

Decluttering is an essential step in creating a minimalist home that supports your well-being and reflects your values. By understanding the benefits of decluttering, exploring various decluttering techniques, and creating a personalized decluttering plan, you'll be well-equipped to tackle the excess in your home and create a living space that brings you joy and peace.

In the next section, we'll dive into a room-by-room decluttering guide, providing specific strategies and tips for simplifying each area of your home. With a solid foundation in the art of decluttering and a clear plan in place, you'll be ready to transform your living space and embrace the benefits of a minimalist lifestyle.

# Room-by-Room Decluttering Guide

Now that you have a solid understanding of the art of decluttering and have created a personalized decluttering plan, it's time to dive into the specifics of simplifying each area of your home. In this section, we'll provide a room-by-room decluttering guide, offering strategies and tips for tackling the living room, kitchen, bedroom, bathroom, home office, and storage spaces.

Living Room

The living room is often the heart of the home, where family members gather to relax, entertain, and spend time together. To create a minimalist living room that promotes comfort and connection, consider the following decluttering strategies:

1. Evaluate furniture: Assess each piece of furniture in your living room and consider its purpose, functionality, and aesthetic value. Remove any items that are rarely used, in disrepair, or no longer align with your style or needs.

2. Simplify decor: Curate a minimalist decor scheme by keeping only those items that hold significant meaning or add value to the space. Remove excess knock-knacks, decorative pillows, and wall art that clutters the room or detracts from a sense of calm.

3. Streamline media and electronics: Declutter your media collection by

digitizing movies, music, and books, and donating or selling physical copies. Organize electronic devices and cords using cable management solutions and designated storage areas.

4. Create multi-functional spaces: Maximize the functionality of your living room by incorporating multi-purpose furniture, such as a storage ottoman or a convertible sofa. These items help reduce clutter by serving multiple needs in a single piece.

5. Establish a regular tidying routine: Maintain a clutter-free living room by establishing a regular tidying routine, such as dedicating 10 minutes each evening to returning items to their designated homes and clearing surfaces.

Kitchen

The kitchen is a high-traffic area prone to clutter and accumulation. To create a minimalist kitchen that is both functional and visually appealing, consider the following decluttering strategies:

1. Declutter cabinets and drawers: Go through each cabinet and drawer, removing duplicate items, unused gadgets, and expired food. Keep only those items that you use regularly and that support your cooking and meal preparation needs.

2. Simplify counter tops: Keep counter tops clear and clutter-free by storing appliances and tools in designated cabinets or drawers. Reserve counter space for frequently used items and those that bring you joy, such as a beautiful tea kettle or a cherished cookbook.

3. Organize the pantry: Declutter your pantry by removing expired items, consolidating similar products, and using clear storage containers to maximize space and visibility. Implement a system for labeling and organizing food items to streamline meal planning and grocery shopping.

4. Curate a minimalist dish and utensil collection: Evaluate your dish and utensil collection, keeping only those items that you use regularly and that serve a specific purpose. Consider donating or re-purposing excess or rarely used items.

5. Embrace open shelving: Consider replacing some upper cabinets with open shelving to showcase a curated collection of dishes, glassware, and kitchen essentials. This approach encourages intersectionality in your possessions and creates a visually appealing, minimalist aesthetic.

Bedroom

The bedroom should be a peaceful sanctuary that promotes relaxation and rest. To create a minimalist bedroom that supports your well-being, consider the following decluttering strategies:

1. Simplify your wardrobe: Declutter your closet by removing clothing items that no longer fit, are in disrepair, or don't align with your current style or lifestyle. Keep only those pieces that you love, wear regularly, and make you feel confident.

2. Minimize bedside clutter: Keep bedside tables clutter-free by storing only essential items, such as a lamp, a book, and a glass of water. Use drawer organizers or small boxes to corral items and maintain a tidy surface.

3. Streamline furniture: Evaluate your bedroom furniture and remove any pieces that are unnecessary or overcrowd the space. Consider investing in multi-functional furniture, such as a bed with built-in storage, to maximize space and reduce clutter.

4. Curate a calming decor scheme: Create a minimalist bedroom decor scheme that promotes relaxation and tranquility. Choose a neutral color palette, incorporate natural elements, and display only those items that bring

you joy or serve a specific purpose.

5. Establish a regular cleaning routine: Maintain a clutter-free bedroom by establishing a regular cleaning routine, such as dedicating 10 minutes each morning to making the bed, clearing surfaces, and returning items to their designated homes.

Bathroom

The bathroom is a functional space that can quickly become cluttered with toiletries, linens, and personal care items. To create a minimalist bathroom that is both practical and visually appealing, consider the following decluttering strategies:

1. Declutter counter tops and cabinets: Go through your bathroom counter tops and cabinets, removing expired products, duplicate items, and those that you no longer use or need. Keep only the essentials that support your daily hygiene and self-care routines.

2. Simplify your toiletry collection: Streamline your toiletry collection by keeping only those products that you use regularly and that align with your personal care needs. Consider investing in multi-purpose products to reduce the overall number of items in your bathroom.

3. Organize linens and towels: Declutter your linen closet by removing worn or stained towels, washcloths, and bedding. Keep only those items that are in good condition and that you use regularly. Consider implementing a rotation system to ensure even wear and tear.

4. Utilize vertical storage: Maximize space in your bathroom by utilizing vertical storage solutions, such as wall-mounted shelves, over-the-door organizers, and hanging baskets. These tools help keep items organized and easily accessible while reducing clutter on counter tops and in cabinets.

5. Embrace minimalist decor: Create a minimalist bathroom aesthetic by choosing a simple color scheme, incorporating natural elements, and displaying only a few carefully curated decor items, such as a plush bath mat or a beautiful plant.

Home Office

The home office is a space for productivity and focus, but it can easily become overwhelmed by paper clutter, office supplies, and technology. To create a minimalist home office that supports your work and creativity, consider the following decluttering strategies:

1. Digitize paper clutter: Scan and digitize important documents, receipts, and paperwork to reduce physical clutter in your home office. Use a digital filing system to organize and store these items securely.

2. Simplify your desk: Keep your desk surface clear and clutter-free by storing only the essentials, such as your computer, a notebook, and a few pens. Use drawer organizers or desk accessories to corral smaller items and maintain a tidy workspace.

3. Curate your book and reference collection: Evaluate your book and reference collection, keeping only those items that you use regularly or that hold significant value. Consider donating or selling books that you have already read or that no longer align with your interests or needs.

4. Streamline technology and cords: Declutter your technology collection by removing outdated or unused devices. Use cable management solutions to organize and conceal cords, creating a visually appealing and clutter-free workspace.

5. Create a minimalist storage system: Implement a minimalist storage system in your home office using a combination of open shelving, file cabinets, and

storage boxes. Label each container clearly and establish a regular routine for returning items to their designated homes.

Storage Spaces

Storage spaces, such as closets, attics, and garages, can quickly become catch-all areas for clutter and unused items. To create minimalist storage spaces that are both functional and organized, consider the following decluttering strategies:

1. Evaluate stored items: Go through each storage space, evaluating the items you have stored. Remove anything that is broken, outdated, or no longer serves a purpose in your life. Be honest about the likelihood of using or needing these items in the future.

2. Categorize and containerize: Group similar items together and store them in clear, labeled containers. This approach makes it easy to find what you need and maintain an organized storage system over time.

3. Maximize vertical space: Utilize vertical space in your storage areas by installing shelving units, hanging organizers, and pegboards. These tools help keep items off the floor and make the most of the available space.

4. Implement a regular review process: Establish a regular review process for your storage spaces, such as dedicating a weekend each season to reassessing and decluttering stored items. This ongoing maintenance helps prevent the accumulation of clutter over time.

5. Consider alternative storage solutions: If your storage spaces are limited or consistently overcrowded, consider alternative storage solutions, such as renting a small storage unit or utilizing off-site document storage for rarely accessed paperwork.

Remember, decluttering is an ongoing process that requires regular maintenance and attention. As you work through each room in your home, be patient with yourself and celebrate the progress you make along the way. By breaking the process down into manageable steps and focusing on one area at a time, you'll soon experience the joys and benefits of a minimalist home that supports your well-being and reflects your values.

As you continue on your minimalist journey, consider exploring the next section on dealing with specific types of items, such as sentimental possessions, paper clutter, and hobby supplies. With a room-by-room decluttering plan in place and a growing understanding of the art of letting go, you'll be well-equipped to navigate the challenges and rewards of creating a minimalist home that truly serves you.

# Dealing with Specific Items

While the room-by-room decluttering guide provides a comprehensive framework for simplifying your living space, certain items can pose unique challenges and require specific strategies for decluttering. In this section, we'll explore how to deal with clothes and accessories, books and papers, electronics and gadgets, and gifts and memorabilia. By addressing these common clutter culprits, you'll be better equipped to create a minimalist home that supports your values and lifestyle.

Clothes and Accessories

Clothing and accessories can quickly accumulate, leading to overstuffed closets and drawers. To create a minimalist wardrobe that is both functional and stylish, consider the following decluttering strategies:

1. Evaluate each item: Go through your clothing and accessories one by one, asking yourself the following questions:
   - Does this item fit well and make me feel confident?
   - Have I worn this item in the past year?
   - Does this item align with my current lifestyle and personal style?
   - Is this item in good condition, or does it require repair or replacement?

If an item doesn't meet these criteria, consider donating, selling, or repurposing it.

2. Create a capsule wardrobe: A capsule wardrobe is a curated collection of versatile, high-quality pieces that can be mixed and matched to create a variety of outfits. By focusing on timeless, well-made items that align with your personal style, you can simplify your wardrobe and reduce the need for excess clothing.

3. Implement the "one-in-one-out" rule: To maintain a minimalist wardrobe over time, consider implementing the "one-in-one-out" rule. For every new clothing or accessory item you bring into your home, commit to removing one item in the same category. This approach helps prevent the accumulation of clutter and encourages intentional consumption.

4. Store clothes strategically: Maximize space and visibility in your closet and drawers by using slim hangers, drawer organizers, and storage boxes. Arrange clothing by category, color, or occasion to make items easy to find and maintain a tidy appearance.

5. Conduct regular reviews: Establish a regular review process for your wardrobe, such as dedicating a weekend each season to reassessing your clothing and accessories. This ongoing maintenance helps ensure that your wardrobe remains aligned with your current needs and style preferences.

Books and Papers

Books and papers can hold sentimental value and intellectual significance, making them challenging to declutter. To create a minimalist library and paper management system, consider the following decluttering strategies:

1. Digitize when possible: Scan and digitize important documents, receipts, and paperwork to reduce physical clutter in your home. Use a digital filing system to organize and store these items securely, making them easily accessible when needed.

2. Evaluate your book collection: Go through your book collection, asking yourself the following questions:
    - Have I read this book, and is it likely that I will re-read it in the future?
    - Does this book hold significant sentimental or intellectual value?
    - Is this book readily available through a library or digital platform?
    - Does this book align with my current interests and goals?

If a book doesn't meet these criteria, consider donating, selling, or gifting it to someone who may appreciate it.

3. Implement a borrowing-first approach: Before purchasing a new book, consider borrowing it from a library or friend first. This approach allows you to enjoy the book without adding to your physical collection and helps you make more intentional purchasing decisions.

4. Create a designated paper processing area: Establish a designated area in your home for processing incoming paper, such as a tray or folder on your desk. Make it a habit to sort through this area regularly, filing important documents and recycling or shredding unneeded papers.

5. Utilize vertical storage: Maximize space and visual appeal in your minimalist library by utilizing vertical storage solutions, such as floating shelves or a slim bookcase. Arrange books by color, size, or genre to create a cohesive and intentional display.

Electronics and Gadgets

Electronics and gadgets can quickly become outdated, leading to a collection of unused devices and tangled cords. To create a minimalist technology setup that is both functional and clutter-free, consider the following decluttering strategies:

1. Evaluate your devices: Go through your electronics and gadgets, asking

yourself the following questions:
  - Do I use this device regularly, or has it been sitting unused for an extended period?
  - Does this device serve a unique purpose, or do I have other devices that can fulfill the same function?
  - Is this device in good working condition, or does it require repair or replacement?
  - Does this device align with my current needs and lifestyle?

If a device doesn't meet these criteria, consider donating, selling, or recycling it responsibly.

2. Consolidate and simplify: Look for opportunities to consolidate your electronics and simplify your setup. For example, consider using a multi-function printer instead of separate devices for printing, scanning, and copying. Or, opt for a single smart device that can fulfill multiple needs, such as a tablet that doubles as an e-reader.

3. Implement cable management solutions: Tame cord clutter by implementing cable management solutions, such as cord organizers, cable ties, or a designated charging station. By keeping cords organized and concealed, you can create a cleaner, more visually appealing technology setup.

4. Embrace cloud storage: Reduce physical clutter associated with electronic media, such as CDs and DVDs, by embracing cloud storage solutions. Digitize your music, movies, and photos, and store them securely in the cloud for easy access from any device.

5. Establish a regular review process: Implement a regular review process for your electronics and gadgets, such as dedicating a weekend each year to reassessing your devices and their functionality. This ongoing maintenance helps ensure that your technology setup remains streamlined and aligned with your current needs.

Gifts and Memorabilia

Gifts and memorabilia can hold deep sentimental value, making them emotionally challenging to declutter. To create a minimalist approach to managing these items, consider the following decluttering strategies:

1. Evaluate the sentiment: Go through your gifts and memorabilia, asking yourself the following questions:
    - Does this item evoke strong positive emotions and memories?
    - Is this item a true representation of the relationship or experience it represents?
    - Can I honor the sentiment behind this item in a way that doesn't involve keeping the physical object?
    - Does displaying or storing this item align with my current values and aesthetic preferences?

If an item doesn't meet these criteria, consider letting it go with gratitude for the role it has played in your life.

2. Take photographs: Before letting go of a sentimental item, consider taking a photograph of it to preserve the memory. Create a digital album or scrapbook of these images, allowing you to reminisce without the physical clutter.

3. Create a designated display space: Designate a specific area in your home, such as a single shelf or shadow box, for displaying a curated selection of your most cherished gifts and memorabilia. By limiting the space available, you encourage yourself to be intentional about which items you choose to keep and honor.

4. Re-purpose or up cycle: Look for opportunities to repurposed or up cycle sentimental items in a way that aligns with your current lifestyle and aesthetic preferences. For example, transform a collection of beloved t-shirts into a cozy quilt, or use a sentimental piece of jewelry as a unique bookmark.

5. Practice gratitude and letting go: As you declutter your gifts and memorabilia, practice gratitude for the love, experiences, and relationships they represent. Acknowledge that letting go of the physical item does not diminish the significance of the sentiment behind it, and trust that the memories will remain even as the object is released.

Remember, decluttering specific items is a deeply personal process that requires patience, self-compassion, and a willingness to let go. By approaching these common clutter culprits with intersectionality and a focus on your values and goals, you can create a minimalist home that truly serves and supports you.

As you continue on your minimalist journey, consider exploring the next section on maintaining your minimalist home over time. With strategies for dealing with specific items and a growing understanding of the art of intentional living, you'll be well-equipped to create a lasting and meaningful minimalist lifestyle.

Once you've decluttered your living space and pared down your possessions to those that truly serve and support you, it's time to focus on designing your minimalist home. Minimalist design is characterized by simplicity, functionality, and a focus on the essential. By incorporating these principles into your living space, you can create a home that is both visually appealing and conducive to a minimalist lifestyle.

# Principles of Minimalist Design

I n this section, we'll explore the core principles of minimalist design, including simplicity, functionality, and aesthetics. We'll also discuss strategies for choosing a color palette that promotes a sense of calm and cohesion, and ways to incorporate natural elements into your minimalist home.

Simplicity, Functionality, and Aesthetics

At the heart of minimalist design are three core principles: simplicity, functionality, and aesthetics. By understanding and embracing these principles, you can create a living space that embodies the essence of minimalism and supports your minimalist lifestyle.

1. Simplicity:
   Simplicity is the foundation of minimalist design. It involves stripping away the unnecessary and focusing on the essential elements of a space. In a minimalist home, simplicity is reflected in the absence of clutter, the streamlined furniture and decor, and the overall sense of openness and breathing room.

To embrace simplicity in your minimalist home, consider the following strategies:
   - Choose furniture and decor with clean lines and simple, geometric shapes.
   - Opt for a limited color palette and avoid busy patterns or excessive

ornamentation.

- Leave ample negative space around furniture and decor to create a sense of openness and flow.

- Edit your possessions regularly, removing items that no longer serve a purpose or align with your minimalist aesthetic.

## 2. Functionality:

Functionality is another key principle of minimalist design. In a minimalist home, every element should serve a purpose and contribute to the overall usability and efficiency of the space. This means choosing furniture and decor that are both beautiful and practical, and arranging them in a way that supports your daily routines and activities.

To prioritize functionality in your minimalist home, consider the following strategies:

- Opt for multi-functional furniture, such as a storage ottoman or a dining table that doubles as a workspace.

- Choose durable, high-quality materials that can withstand daily wear and tear.

- Arrange furniture to create distinct zones for different activities, such as relaxing, working, or dining.

- Consider the flow and circulation of the space, ensuring that there is ample room to move around and access essential items.

## 3. Aesthetics:

While simplicity and functionality are essential, minimalist design is also characterized by a strong sense of aesthetics. A minimalist home should be visually pleasing and cohesive, with a carefully curated selection of furniture, decor, and finishes that work together to create a sense of harmony and balance.

To create a strong aesthetic in your minimalist home, consider the following strategies:

- Choose a cohesive color palette and stick to it throughout the space.

- Opt for high-quality, timeless pieces that will endure both physically and stylistically.

- Incorporate texture through natural materials, such as wood, stone, or linen, to add visual interest and depth.

- Display a few carefully chosen pieces of artwork or decor that hold personal meaning or reflect your minimalist values.

By embracing simplicity, functionality, and aesthetics in your minimalist home design, you can create a living space that is both beautiful and practical, and that supports your minimalist lifestyle.

Choosing a Color Palette

Color plays a significant role in minimalist design, setting the tone and atmosphere of a space. A well-chosen color palette can promote a sense of calm, balance, and cohesion, while a poorly chosen palette can create visual chaos and detract from the overall minimalist aesthetic.

When choosing a color palette for your minimalist home, consider the following strategies:

1. Opt for a neutral base:
   A neutral base is the foundation of a minimalist color palette. Neutral colors, such as white, beige, gray, and taupe, create a sense of simplicity and serenity, and provide a versatile backdrop for other design elements. Neutral walls, floors, and larger pieces of furniture establish a cohesive and calming base for your minimalist home.

2. Incorporate accent colors:
   While a neutral base is essential, incorporating accent colors can add visual interest and personality to your minimalist home. Accent colors should be used sparingly and intentionally, typically on smaller pieces of furniture,

decor, or artwork. When selecting accent colors, consider the following tips:

- Choose colors that complement your neutral base and create a sense of harmony and balance.

- Opt for muted or saturated versions of your chosen accent colors to maintain a minimalist aesthetic.

- Use accent colors to highlight specific areas or features of your home, such as a piece of artwork or a cozy reading nook.

3. Consider the mood and atmosphere:

Color has a significant impact on the mood and atmosphere of a space. When choosing a color palette for your minimalist home, consider the desired mood and atmosphere of each room. For example:

- Cool colors, such as blue and green, create a sense of calm and tranquility, making them ideal for bedrooms and bathrooms.

- Warm colors, such as yellow and orange, create a sense of warmth and energy, making them suitable for living rooms and kitchens.

- Neutral colors, such as white and gray, create a sense of simplicity and sophistication, making them appropriate for any room in the home.

4. Embrace tonal variations:

To create visual interest and depth in a minimalist color palette, embrace tonal variations of your chosen colors. This means incorporating different shades, tints, and tones of the same hue throughout your home. For example, you might pair a light beige wall with a slightly darker beige sofa, and accent the space with a few cream-colored pillows. Tonal variations add subtle visual interest without detracting from the overall minimalist aesthetic.

5. Consider the natural light:

The natural light in your home can have a significant impact on how colors appear and how they make you feel. When choosing a color palette for your minimalist home, consider the quality and quantity of natural light in each room. For example:

- In rooms with ample natural light, you can afford to use darker or more saturated colors without making the space feel heavy or claustrophobic.

- In rooms with limited natural light, opt for lighter and brighter colors to help reflect the available light and create a sense of openness and airiness.

By choosing a color palette that promotes simplicity, harmony, and balance, you can create a minimalist home that is both visually appealing and conducive to a peaceful and intentional lifestyle.

Incorporating Natural Elements

Incorporating natural elements into your minimalist home design can help create a sense of warmth, texture, and connection to the outside world. Natural materials and elements also align with the minimalist values of simplicity and sustainability, making them a popular choice in minimalist homes.

When incorporating natural elements into your minimalist home, consider the following strategies:

1. Use natural materials:
   Natural materials, such as wood, stone, linen, and cotton, add warmth, texture, and visual interest to a minimalist home. These materials also age gracefully and develop a unique patina over time, contributing to the overall character and charm of the space. Consider incorporating natural materials in the following ways:

- Use wood flooring, furniture, or accents to add warmth and texture to a room.

- Incorporate stone or concrete elements, such as a fireplace surround or a kitchen counter top, to add visual weight and grounding to a space.

- Choose linen or cotton textiles for curtains, bedding, and upholstery to add softness and natural texture to a room.

2. Bring in plants:

Plants are a simple and effective way to incorporate natural elements into your minimalist home. In addition to adding visual interest and texture, plants also help purify the air and create a sense of connection to the natural world. When selecting plants for your minimalist home, consider the following tips:

- Choose plants that thrive in the available light and environmental conditions of each room.

- Opt for plants with simple, sculptural shapes that complement the minimalist aesthetic, such as snake plants, fiddle leaf figs, or rubber trees.

- Use plants to add pops of color and life to a neutral color palette.

- Group plants together in odd numbers to create visual balance and interest.


3. Maximize natural light:

Natural light is a key element in minimalist design, helping to create a sense of openness, airiness, and connection to the outside world. To maximize natural light in your minimalist home, consider the following strategies:

- Use sheer or lightweight curtains to filter light while maintaining privacy.

- Position mirrors opposite windows to reflect and amplify the available natural light.

- Choose light-colored or reflective surfaces, such as white walls or glossy tile, to help bounce light around the space.

- Consider adding skylights or solar tubes to bring natural light into darker or interior rooms.


4. Incorporate natural textures:

In addition to natural materials, incorporating natural textures can help add visual interest and depth to a minimalist home. Natural textures, such as woven baskets, jute rugs, or driftwood accents, add a sense of warmth and organic character to a space. When incorporating natural textures into your minimalist home, consider the following tips:

- Choose textures that complement the overall color palette and aesthetic of the space.

- Use natural textures sparingly and intentionally to avoid overwhelming the minimalist design.

- Mix and match different textures to create visual interest and contrast, such as pairing a smooth stone vase with a rough-hewn wooden tray.

5. Embrace biophilic design:

Biophilic design is a concept that seeks to integrate nature and natural elements into the built environment to promote health, well-being, and a sense of connection to the natural world. To embrace biophilic design in your minimalist home, consider the following strategies:

- Incorporate natural materials, plants, and textures throughout the space.
- Maximize natural light and views of the outdoors, using windows, skylights, and glass doors to blur the boundaries between inside and out.
- Use nature-inspired colors, patterns, and motifs in artwork, textiles, and decor.
- Create indoor-outdoor connections, such as a balcony or patio, to extend your living space and embrace the natural world.

By incorporating natural elements into your minimalist home design, you can create a living space that is both visually appealing and conducive to a sense of well-being and connection to the natural world. Natural materials, plants, light, and textures all contribute to a warm, inviting, and peaceful minimalist home.

As you continue on your minimalist journey, consider exploring the next section on furniture and decor for your minimalist home. With a strong foundation in the principles of minimalist design and a growing understanding of how to incorporate natural elements, you'll be well-equipped to create a beautiful and functional minimalist living space that truly reflects your values and lifestyle.

# Furniture and Decor

Furniture and decor play a crucial role in creating a minimalist home that is both functional and visually appealing. In a minimalist space, each piece of furniture and decor should be carefully chosen for its purpose, quality, and aesthetic value. By selecting essential furniture pieces, incorporating minimalist decor ideas, and creating multi-functional spaces, you can design a home that embodies the principles of minimalism and supports your lifestyle.

In this section, we'll explore strategies for selecting essential furniture pieces that are both functional and beautiful, minimalist decor ideas that add character and interest to your space, and ways to create multi-functional spaces that maximize the efficiency and flexibility of your home.

Selecting Essential Furniture Pieces

When selecting furniture for your minimalist home, it's important to focus on pieces that are essential to your daily life and that contribute to the overall functionality and aesthetic of your space. By carefully curating your furniture collection, you can create a home that is both comfortable and visually appealing, without unnecessary clutter or excess.

Here are some key considerations when selecting essential furniture pieces for your minimalist home:

1. Prioritize functionality: Each piece of furniture in your minimalist home should serve a clear purpose and contribute to the overall functionality of your space. Before making a purchase, consider how the piece will be used and whether it meets your specific needs and requirements. For example, a comfortable sofa that can accommodate your family and guests, or a dining table that can double as a workspace, are essential pieces that prioritize functionality.

2. Invest in quality: In a minimalist home, each piece of furniture is given more visual attention and is likely to receive more wear and tear due to its frequent use. Investing in high-quality, durable furniture ensures that your pieces will stand the test of time, both physically and aesthetically. Look for furniture made from sturdy materials, with strong construction and timeless design, to ensure that your investment will last for years to come.

3. Choose versatile pieces: Versatile furniture pieces that can serve multiple purposes are essential in a minimalist home. Look for pieces that can be used in different ways or that can adapt to changing needs, such as a modular sofa that can be reconfigured for different seating arrangements, or a coffee table with hidden storage compartments. Versatile furniture allows you to maximize the functionality of your space while minimizing the number of pieces you need to own.

4. Opt for timeless design: When selecting furniture for your minimalist home, opt for pieces with timeless design that will remain stylish and relevant for years to come. Classic shapes, neutral colors, and simple, clean lines are all hallmarks of timeless furniture design. By choosing pieces that are not tied to current trends or fads, you can create a minimalist space that feels both contemporary and enduring.

5. Consider size and scale: The size and scale of your furniture pieces are important considerations in a minimalist home. Opt for furniture that is proportional to the size of your space, and that allows for easy movement

and flow. In smaller spaces, consider using furniture with slim profiles or transparent materials, such as glass or acrylic, to maintain a sense of openness and airiness. In larger spaces, use furniture to define distinct zones and create a sense of intimacy and coziness.

6. Embrace negative space: In a minimalist home, the space around your furniture is just as important as the furniture itself. Embrace negative space by leaving ample room around each piece of furniture, and by choosing pieces with clean, simple lines that don't overwhelm the space. By allowing your furniture to breathe, you create a sense of openness and tranquility that is essential to the minimalist aesthetic.

By selecting essential furniture pieces that prioritize functionality, quality, versatility, timeless design, size and scale, and negative space, you can create a minimalist home that is both comfortable and visually appealing. Remember, the goal is not to have as few pieces of furniture as possible, but rather to curate a collection of essential pieces that truly support and enhance your lifestyle.

Minimalist Decor Ideas

In a minimalist home, decor is used sparingly and intentionally to add character, texture, and visual interest to the space. Rather than filling every surface with knick-knacks and hopscotches, minimalist decor is carefully curated to complement the overall aesthetic and create a sense of harmony and balance.

Here are some minimalist decor ideas to help you add personality and style to your space:

1. Incorporate natural elements: Natural elements, such as plants, wood, stone, and natural fibers, add warmth, texture, and visual interest to a minimalist space. Consider incorporating a few carefully chosen plants,

such as a sculptural succulent or a leafy fig tree, to bring life and energy to your home. Use natural materials, such as a wooden bowl or a stone vase, to add organic texture and visual depth.

2. Use artwork as a focal point: In a minimalist home, artwork is often used as a focal point to add personality and character to the space. Choose one or two large-scale pieces that reflect your personal style and complement the overall color palette and aesthetic of your home. Hang artwork at eye level and allow plenty of negative space around each piece to maintain a sense of openness and simplicity.

3. Display meaningful objects: While minimalist decor is intentionally sparse, it's important to include a few meaningful objects that reflect your personality and values. Choose objects that hold sentimental value or that tell a story, such as a cherished family heirloom or a piece of art from a memorable trip. Display these objects intentionally, using them to create visual interest and to spark conversation.

4. Embrace texture: Texture is an important element in minimalist decor, adding visual interest and depth to a simple, pared-down space. Incorporate texture through natural materials, such as a chunky knit throw blanket or a woven jute rug, or through subtle patterns, such as a hand-printed fabric or a marbled ceramic vase. By layering different textures, you create a sense of warmth and dimension that keeps the space from feeling cold or sterile.

5. Use color intentionally: In a minimalist home, color is used intentionally and sparingly to create visual interest and to evoke a specific mood or atmosphere. Choose a neutral base color palette, such as white, gray, or beige, and add pops of color through artwork, textiles, or accent pieces. Use color to highlight specific areas or features of your home, such as a bold piece of art or a colorful throw pillow, while keeping the overall palette simple and cohesive.

6. Incorporate negative space: Just as with furniture, negative space is an important element in minimalist decor. Allow plenty of empty space around each decor item, and resist the urge to fill every surface or corner with objects. By embracing negative space, you create a sense of openness and tranquility that allows each decor item to shine and that keeps the overall space from feeling cluttered or overwhelming.

7. Choose functional decor: In a minimalist home, decor should be both beautiful and functional. Look for decor items that serve a specific purpose, such as a set of nesting bowls that can be used for storage or serving, or a sculptural vase that doubles as a bookend. By choosing decor that is both aesthetically pleasing and practical, you maximize the efficiency and functionality of your space while maintaining a minimalist aesthetic.

By incorporating these minimalist decor ideas into your home, you can add personality, character, and visual interest to your space while maintaining a sense of simplicity and intention. Remember, the key is to choose decor items sparingly and intentionally, and to allow each item room to breathe and shine.

Creating Multi-Functional Spaces

In a minimalist home, creating multi-functional spaces is essential to maximizing the efficiency and flexibility of your living area. By designing rooms that can serve multiple purposes and by choosing furniture that can adapt to different needs, you can make the most of your square footage and create a home that is both functional and versatile.

Here are some strategies for creating multi-functional spaces in your minimalist home:

1. Define zones within a room: One way to create a multi-functional space is to define distinct zones within a single room, each serving a specific purpose.

For example, in a small studio apartment, you might create a sleeping zone with a bed and nightstand, a dining zone with a table and chairs, and a living zone with a sofa and coffee table. By using furniture and decor to define these zones, you can create a sense of separation and purpose within an open-concept space.

2. Use furniture that serves multiple purposes: Another strategy for creating multi-functional spaces is to choose furniture that can serve multiple purposes or that can adapt to different needs. For example, a dining table that can double as a workspace, a coffee table with hidden storage compartments, or a sofa bed that can accommodate overnight guests. By investing in versatile furniture pieces, you can maximize the functionality of your space without adding unnecessary clutter.

3. Incorporate flexible seating: Flexible seating options, such as floor cushions, poufs, or stack able stools, can help you create a multi-functional space that can adapt to different needs and occasions. These seating options can be easily moved or stored away when not in use, allowing you to reconfigure your space as needed. For example, floor cushions can provide extra seating for guests during a party, or can be used as a cozy reading nook in a corner of your living room.

4. Maximize vertical space: In a minimalist home, maximizing vertical space is key to creating multi-functional spaces that are both efficient and organized. Use wall-mounted shelves, hanging organizers, or vertical storage systems to make the most of your wall space and to keep items off the floor. For example, a wall-mounted desk can double as a workspace and a dining table, while a hanging organizer can store kitchen tools or office supplies.

5. Use room dividers: Room dividers, such as screens, curtains, or book-shelves, can help you create multi-functional spaces by separating different areas of a room or by providing privacy and sound insulation. For example, a bookshelf can serve as a room divider between a living area and a home office,

while a curtain can separate a sleeping area from a living area in a studio apartment. By using room dividers strategically, you can create distinct zones within a single space, each serving a specific purpose.

6. Incorporate hidden storage: Hidden storage solutions, such as under-bed drawers, ottoman coffee tables, or wall-mounted cabinets, can help you create multi-functional spaces by maximizing storage while minimizing clutter. By keeping items out of sight but easily accessible, you can maintain a minimalist aesthetic while still having everything you need close at hand. For example, a bed with built-in storage drawers can provide extra space for linens or seasonal clothing, while a wall-mounted cabinet can store office supplies or media equipment.

7. Embrace convertible spaces: Convertible spaces, such as a home office that can be transformed into a guest room or a dining room that can be used as a playroom, are the ultimate multi-functional solution. By using furniture that can be easily moved or reconfigured, such as a Murphy bed or a folding table, you can create spaces that can adapt to different needs and occasions. Embracing convertible spaces allows you to maximize the flexibility and efficiency of your home, while still maintaining a minimalist aesthetic.

By creating multi-functional spaces in your minimalist home, you can maximize the efficiency and flexibility of your living area, while still maintaining a sense of simplicity and intention. Remember, the key is to choose furniture and decor that can adapt to different needs, and to use space strategically to create distinct zones and purposes within a single room.

As you continue on your minimalist journey, consider exploring the next section on organization and storage solutions for your minimalist home. With a strong foundation in furniture selection, decor ideas, and multi-functional space design, you'll be well-equipped to create a home that is both beautiful and practical, and that truly supports your minimalist lifestyle.

# Organization and Storage Solutions

In a minimalist home, effective organization and storage solutions are essential to maintaining a clutter-free and functional living space. By maximizing storage potential, incorporating creative storage ideas, and implementing strategies for maintaining a tidy home, you can create a peaceful and efficient environment that supports your minimalist lifestyle.

In this section, we'll explore various ways to maximize storage in a minimalist home, share creative storage ideas that are both functional and aesthetically pleasing, and provide tips for maintaining a clutter-free space over time.

Maximizing Storage in a Minimalist Home

One of the key challenges in a minimalist home is finding ways to store necessary items without compromising the clean, uncluttered aesthetic. By maximizing storage potential in every room, you can ensure that your belongings have a designated place and that your living space remains organized and visually appealing.

Here are some strategies for maximizing storage in a minimalist home:

1. Utilize vertical space: In a minimalist home, making use of vertical space is crucial to maximizing storage potential. Install shelving units that extend from floor to ceiling, hang organizers on the back of doors, and use wall-mounted storage solutions to keep items off the floor and easily accessible.

By taking advantage of the often-overlooked vertical space in your home, you can significantly increase your storage capacity without sacrificing square footage.

2. Invest in multi-functional furniture: When selecting furniture for your minimalist home, look for pieces that serve multiple purposes and offer built-in storage solutions. For example, a bed with drawers underneath, a coffee table with hidden compartments, or a bench with a lift-up seat for storing blankets and pillows. By choosing furniture that doubles as storage, you can maximize the functionality of your space and keep clutter at bay.

3. Make use of awkward spaces: Every home has awkward spaces that are often overlooked or underutilized, such as the area under a staircase, the gap between the refrigerator and the wall, or the space above a doorway. By getting creative with your storage solutions, you can turn these awkward spaces into valuable storage areas. Consider installing custom shelving, using tension rods to create hanging storage, or adding a slim rolling cart to maximize these often-wasted spaces.

4. Implement a "one in, one out" policy: To maintain a clutter-free home and avoid the need for additional storage, consider implementing a "one in, one out" policy. This means that for every new item you bring into your home, you commit to removing one item in the same category. By following this rule, you can ensure that your belongings remain manageable and that your storage solutions continue to meet your needs over time.

5. Regularly reassess and declutter: Even with the best storage solutions in place, clutter can still accumulate over time. To maximize storage potential in your minimalist home, it's important to regularly reassess your belongings and declutter as needed. Set aside time each season to go through your possessions, evaluating what you truly need and use, and letting go of items that no longer serve you. By maintaining a regular decluttering practice, you can ensure that your storage solutions remain effective and that your home

stays organized and clutter-free.

By implementing these strategies for maximizing storage potential, you can create a minimalist home that is both functional and visually appealing. Remember, the key is to be intentional with your belongings and to make the most of every available space in your home.

Creative Storage Ideas

In addition to maximizing storage potential through strategic organization and multi-functional furniture, incorporating creative storage ideas can help you maintain a clutter-free and visually appealing minimalist home. By thinking outside the box and utilizing unconventional storage solutions, you can keep your belongings organized and easily accessible while adding a touch of personality and style to your space.

Here are some creative storage ideas to inspire your minimalist home:

1. Hanging storage: Hanging storage solutions are a great way to maximize vertical space and keep items off the floor. Consider using hanging organizers for storing shoes, bags, or accessories, or installing a pegboard in your home office or craft room for keeping tools and supplies within easy reach. You can also use hanging baskets or planters to store items like toiletries, kitchen essentials, or even small plants.

2. Mason jars and clear containers: Mason jars and clear containers are not only visually appealing but also incredibly versatile storage solutions. Use them to store dry goods in your pantry, organize office supplies on your desk, or keep bathroom essentials like cotton balls and Q-tips easily accessible. The clear material allows you to quickly see what's inside, making it easy to find what you need and maintain a tidy appearance.

3. Magnetic knife strip: A magnetic knife strip is a great alternative to a bulky

knife block, freeing up valuable counter space in your kitchen. But this clever storage solution isn't just for knives – you can also use it to store other metal items like scissors, tweezers, or even small jars of spices. Mount a magnetic strip on the wall or inside a cabinet door for a creative and space-saving storage solution.

4. Over-the-door organizers: Over-the-door organizers are a simple and effective way to maximize storage space in any room. Use them to store cleaning supplies in your utility closet, organize jewelry and accessories in your bedroom, or keep scarves and hats easily accessible in your entryway. These organizers come in a variety of styles and sizes, making it easy to find one that fits your specific needs and aesthetic preferences.

5. Tension rods: Tension rods are an inexpensive and versatile storage solution that can be used in a variety of ways throughout your home. Install them vertically in a cabinet to create customized shelving for storing baking sheets or cutting boards, or use them horizontally to hang cleaning supplies or even shoes in your closet. You can also use tension rods to create a makeshift drying rack in your laundry room or to hang curtains for concealing storage areas.

6. Wall-mounted file folders: Wall-mounted file folders are a great way to keep important documents and papers organized and easily accessible without taking up valuable desk or drawer space. Use them in your home office to store bills, contracts, or other important papers, or in your kitchen to keep recipe cards and meal planning documents at hand. You can also use wall-mounted file folders in your entryway to store mail and other incoming papers.

7. Rolling carts: Rolling carts are a versatile and mobile storage solution that can be used in a variety of ways throughout your home. Use them in your kitchen to store frequently used appliances or ingredients, in your bathroom to organize toiletries and linens, or in your home office to keep craft supplies

or project materials easily accessible. The wheels allow you to move the cart as needed, making it easy to adapt to your changing storage needs.

By incorporating these creative storage ideas into your minimalist home, you can keep your belongings organized and easily accessible while adding a touch of personality and style to your space. Remember, the key is to think outside the box and look for unconventional solutions that work for your specific needs and aesthetic preferences.

Maintaining a Clutter-Free Space

Once you've maximized storage potential and incorporated creative storage solutions into your minimalist home, the next challenge is maintaining a clutter-free space over time. Even with the best intentions and systems in place, clutter can still accumulate if you're not proactive about keeping it at bay.

Here are some strategies for maintaining a clutter-free space in your minimalist home:

1. Develop a daily tidying habit: One of the most effective ways to maintain a clutter-free space is to develop a daily tidying habit. This means taking a few minutes each day to put items back in their designated places, wipe down surfaces, and generally tidy up your living space. By making tidying a daily practice, you can prevent clutter from accumulating and keep your home looking and feeling organized and peaceful.

2. Follow the "one-minute rule": The "one-minute rule" is a simple but powerful strategy for maintaining a clutter-free space. The idea is that if a task takes less than one minute to complete, you do it right away rather than putting it off for later. This might include hanging up your coat when you walk in the door, putting your dishes in the dishwasher after a meal, or filing a piece of mail as soon as you've opened it. By taking care of these

small tasks immediately, you can prevent them from piling up and becoming overwhelming.

3. Create designated "landing spots": Another way to maintain a clutter-free space is to create designated "landing spots" for items that tend to accumulate, such as mail, keys, or shoes. By having a specific place for these items to go as soon as you enter your home, you can prevent them from ending up scattered throughout your living space. Consider using a tray or basket near your entryway for keys and mail, and installing a shoe rack or cubby for keeping footwear organized.

4. Use labels and containers: Labeling storage containers and shelves can help you maintain a clutter-free space by making it easy to find what you need and put items back in their designated places. Use clear containers or bins with labels to organize items in your pantry, closet, or home office, and consider using a label maker or chalkboard labels for a clean and cohesive look. By making it easy to see what goes where, you can encourage yourself and others in your household to maintain an organized and clutter-free space.

5. Implement a "re-homing" schedule: Even with regular decluttering, some items may linger in your home unused, taking up valuable space and contributing to visual clutter. To combat this, consider implementing a "re-homing" schedule for items that you're unsure about keeping. For example, if you have a piece of clothing that you haven't worn in six months, put it in a designated box or bag and make a note to revisit it in another three months. If you still haven't worn it at that point, it's likely time to let it go.

6. Make decluttering a family affair: If you share your home with others, maintaining a clutter-free space can be a challenge if everyone isn't on board. To help encourage a household-wide commitment to minimalism, make decluttering a family affair. Schedule regular decluttering sessions where everyone goes through their own belongings and decides what to keep, donate, or discard. You can also assign specific tasks or areas to each family member

to help distribute the workload and ensure that everyone is contributing to the overall organization of your home.

7. Celebrate your progress: Finally, don't forget to celebrate your progress as you work to maintain a clutter-free space in your minimalist home. Recognize the hard work and dedication that goes into keeping your living space organized and uncluttered, and take time to enjoy the peace and calm that comes with a minimalist lifestyle. By acknowledging your successes and the positive impact that minimalism has on your life, you can stay motivated to maintain a clutter-free space over the long term.

By implementing these strategies for maintaining a clutter-free space, you can ensure that your minimalist home remains organized, functional, and visually appealing over time. Remember, the key is to develop consistent habits and systems that work for you and your household, and to approach minimalism as an ongoing practice rather than a one-time event.

As you continue on your minimalist journey, consider exploring the next section on embracing a minimalist lifestyle beyond the home. With a strong foundation in organization and storage solutions, you'll be well-equipped to extend the principles of minimalism to other areas of your life, from your wardrobe and digital presence to your daily routines and overall mindset

# Adopting a Minimalist Lifestyle

M inimalism is more than just a design aesthetic or a way to organize your home – it's a lifestyle that permeates all aspects of your life. By adopting a minimalist mindset and applying its principles to areas beyond your physical space, you can cultivate a more intentional, fulfilling, and sustainable way of living.

In this section, we'll explore what it means to embrace minimalism beyond the home, including how to apply minimalist principles to your consumption habits, relationships, and digital life. We'll also discuss the connection between minimalism and sustainable and ethical living, and provide strategies for adopting a more environmentally conscious lifestyle. Finally, we'll delve into the concept of digital minimalism and offer tips for decluttering your digital space and cultivating a healthier relationship with technology.

Minimalism Beyond the Home

While decluttering and organizing your physical space is a crucial aspect of minimalism, the philosophy extends far beyond the walls of your home. Embracing minimalism as a lifestyle means applying its principles to all areas of your life, from your relationships and work to your hobbies and personal growth.

Here are some ways to embrace minimalism beyond the home:

1. Simplify your schedule: Just as you declutter your physical space, look for ways to declutter your schedule and simplify your commitments. Evaluate how you spend your time and energy, and identify activities or obligations that no longer serve you or align with your values. Be intentional about how you allocate your time, focusing on the people and pursuits that bring you joy and fulfillment.

2. Cultivate meaningful relationships: Minimalism is about quality over quantity, and this extends to your relationships as well. Focus on cultivating deep, meaningful connections with the people who matter most to you, rather than trying to maintain a large network of superficial acquaintances. Be intentional about how you nurture and prioritize your relationships, and don't be afraid to let go of those that drain your energy or bring more stress than joy.

3. Practice mindful consumption: Minimalism encourages a more intentional approach to consumption, both in terms of material possessions and the media you consume. Be mindful of your purchasing habits, and strive to buy only what you truly need or love. Similarly, be selective about the information and entertainment you consume, choosing sources that educate, inspire, or bring you genuine enjoyment.

4. Prioritize experiences over possessions: Rather than seeking fulfillment through material possessions, focus on cultivating meaningful experiences and memories. Invest in travel, learning new skills, or pursuing hobbies that bring you joy and personal growth. By shifting your focus from things to experiences, you can cultivate a richer, more fulfilling life with less emphasis on material possessions.

5. Simplify your finances: Minimalism can also be applied to your financial life, helping you cultivate a more intentional and streamlined approach to money management. Evaluate your spending habits and look for ways to simplify your budget, such as cutting unnecessary expenses or consolidating

accounts. Consider adopting a "less is more" approach to your finances, focusing on saving, investing, and using your money in ways that align with your values and long-term goals.

6. Embrace a growth mindset: Minimalism is not about deprivation or stagnation, but rather about creating space for growth and personal development. Embrace a growth mindset by continually learning, challenging yourself, and seeking out new experiences and perspectives. By letting go of what no longer serves you, you create room for new opportunities and possibilities to enter your life.

By extending the principles of minimalism beyond your physical space, you can cultivate a more intentional, balanced, and fulfilling life. Remember, minimalism is a personal journey, and what it looks like in practice will vary from person to person. The key is to identify what truly matters to you and to align your choices and actions with those values.

Sustainable and Ethical Living

Minimalism and sustainable living are closely intertwined, as both philosophies encourage a more intentional and mindful approach to consumption and resource use. By adopting a minimalist lifestyle, you naturally reduce your environmental impact by buying less, wasting less, and focusing on quality over quantity.

Here are some ways to embrace sustainable and ethical living as part of your minimalist lifestyle:

1. Buy secondhand or Eco-friendly products: When you do need to make a purchase, consider buying secondhand or choosing products made from sustainable, Eco-friendly materials. Buying used items reduces demand for new production and keeps perfectly good items out of landfills. When buying new, look for products with minimal packaging, made from recycled or

biodegradable materials, or certified by reputable environmental organizations.

2. Support ethical and sustainable brands: Do your research and support brands that prioritize ethical labor practices, environmental sustainability, and social responsibility. Look for companies that use sustainable materials, minimize waste and pollution, and treat their workers fairly. By voting with your dollars, you can help create demand for more ethical and sustainable products and practices.

3. Reduce your energy and water consumption: Minimizing your energy and water usage is good for the planet and your wallet. Adopt simple habits like turning off lights when not in use, unplugging electronics, fixing leaky faucets, and taking shorter showers. Consider investing in energy-efficient appliances, installing low-flow fixtures, or exploring renewable energy options like solar panels.

4. Embrace a plant-based diet: Animal agriculture is a significant contributor to greenhouse gas emissions, deforestation, and water pollution. By adopting a plant-based diet or reducing your consumption of animal products, you can significantly reduce your environmental impact. Experiment with meatless meals, buy local and organic produce when possible, and be mindful of the resources that go into your food choices.

5. Minimize waste and properly dispose of items: Strive to minimize waste in your daily life by choosing reusable products over disposables, composting food scraps, and properly recycling or disposing of items that have reached the end of their usefulness. Educate yourself on your local waste management guidelines and look for ways to reduce your overall waste output.

6. Advocate for systemic change: While individual actions are important, true sustainability requires systemic change. Use your voice and your vote to advocate for policies and practices that prioritize environmental protection,

social justice, and ethical business practices. Support organizations and initiatives that are working to create a more sustainable and equitable world.

By integrating sustainable and ethical living practices into your minimalist lifestyle, you can align your values with your actions and contribute to a healthier, more resilient planet. Remember, perfection isn't the goal – even small changes can make a big difference when adopted by many people. Focus on progress over perfection and celebrate the positive impact of your choices.

Digital Minimalism

In today's technology-driven world, our digital lives can be just as cluttered and overwhelming as our physical spaces. From overflowing inboxes to endless social media scrolling, our devices and online presence can be a significant source of distraction and stress. By embracing digital minimalism, you can declutter your digital space, reclaim your time and attention, and cultivate a healthier relationship with technology.

Here are some strategies for embracing digital minimalism:

1. Conduct a digital declutter: Just as you declutter your physical space, periodically conduct a digital declutter to eliminate virtual clutter and streamline your online presence. Unsubscribe from newsletters and mailing lists that no longer serve you, delete unused apps and files, and organize your digital documents and photos into a streamlined filing system.

2. Be intentional with social media: Social media can be a significant time-sink and source of comparison and FOMO (fear of missing out). Be intentional about how you use social media, curating your feeds to include only content that inspires, informs, or brings you joy. Consider taking regular breaks from social media or setting specific boundaries around when and how you engage with these platforms.

3. Minimize notifications and distractions: Constant notifications and alerts can be a major source of distraction and stress. Take control of your digital environment by turning off non-essential notifications, using "Do Not Disturb" mode when focusing on important tasks, and being mindful of how often you check your devices. Consider using apps or browser extensions that block distracting websites or limit your time on certain platforms.

4. Cultivate analog hobbies and activities: Engage in hobbies and activities that don't involve screens or technology, such as reading physical books, practicing a musical instrument, or exploring nature. By cultivating analog pursuits, you give your mind a break from digital stimulation and engage in activities that promote mindfulness, creativity, and relaxation.

5. Create tech-free zones and times: Designate specific areas of your home or times of day as tech-free zones, such as the dinner table or bedroom. Use these tech-free spaces and times to connect with loved ones, engage in self-care practices, or simply be present in the moment without the constant pull of digital distractions.

6. Practice mindful consumption: Be intentional about the digital content you consume, choosing sources that educate, inspire, or bring you genuine value. Avoid mindless scrolling or clicking, and be selective about the information and media you allow into your digital space. Consider setting specific intentions or goals for your online time, rather than getting lost in a sea of endless content.

7. Prioritize real-life connections: While technology can be a valuable tool for staying connected with others, prioritize real-life, face-to-face interactions whenever possible. Make time for in-person conversations, shared meals, and experiences that foster genuine human connection. Remember that digital communication is not a substitute for the depth and richness of real-life relationships.

By adopting a minimalist approach to your digital life, you can reclaim your time, attention, and mental energy for the things that truly matter. Remember, technology is a tool meant to enhance our lives, not control them. By being intentional and mindful about how you engage with digital media and devices, you can cultivate a more balanced and fulfilling relationship with technology.

Embracing minimalism as a lifestyle is an ongoing journey that extends far beyond the walls of your home. By applying minimalist principles to your consumption habits, relationships, and digital life, you can cultivate a more intentional, balanced, and fulfilling existence. Remember, minimalism looks different for everyone – the key is to identify your values and priorities and align your choices and actions accordingly.

As you continue to explore and deepen your minimalist practice, be patient with yourself and celebrate the small wins along the way. Embracing minimalism is not about achieving perfection or adhering to a strict set of rules, but rather about creating space for what truly matters and living in alignment with your values.

In the next section, we'll explore strategies for maintaining your minimalist home and lifestyle over time. With a foundation in the principles of minimalism and a commitment to living intentionally, you'll be well-equipped to navigate the ongoing journey of living minimally and reaping its many benefits.

# Maintaining Your Minimalist Home

Creating a minimalist home is a significant accomplishment, but the journey doesn't end there. Maintaining a clutter-free, intentional living space requires ongoing effort and commitment. Without regular upkeep and a shift in mindset, it's all too easy for clutter to creep back in and for old habits to resurface.

In this section, we'll explore strategies for maintaining your minimalist home over the long term. We'll discuss the importance of establishing routines and habits that support your minimalist lifestyle, introduce the concept of the one-in-one-out rule for managing new possessions, and provide tips for conducting regular decluttering sessions and reassessing your belongings over time. By implementing these strategies, you can ensure that your minimalist home remains a source of peace, clarity, and inspiration for years to come.

Establishing Routines and Habits

One of the keys to maintaining a minimalist home is establishing routines and habits that support your minimalist lifestyle. By incorporating regular decluttering, cleaning, and organizing practices into your daily or weekly schedule, you can prevent clutter from accumulating and keep your living space looking and feeling its best.

Here are some routines and habits to consider implementing:

1. Daily reset: At the end of each day, take a few minutes to tidy up your living space. Put away any items that have been left out, clear surfaces of clutter, and ensure that everything is in its designated place. This daily reset helps prevent clutter from building up over time and allows you to start each day with a clean, organized space.

2. Regular cleaning schedule: Establish a regular cleaning schedule that works for your lifestyle and stick to it. This might involve dedicating certain days of the week to specific tasks, such as vacuuming, dusting, or cleaning bathrooms. By breaking your cleaning routine into manageable chunks and tackling tasks on a consistent basis, you can maintain a tidy, clutter-free home without feeling overwhelmed.

3. Laundry and dish routines: Develop routines for managing laundry and dishes to prevent these items from piling up and creating visual clutter. For example, you might do a load of laundry every few days and put away clean clothes immediately, or make a habit of washing dishes after each meal and putting them away in their designated spots.

4. Paperwork and mail processing: Create a system for processing paperwork and mail on a regular basis to prevent these items from accumulating. This might involve setting aside time each week to sort through mail, pay bills, and file important documents. Consider going paperless whenever possible and unsubscribing from unnecessary mailings to reduce the influx of paper clutter.

5. Seasonal decluttering: In addition to regular decluttering sessions (which we'll discuss in more detail later), consider conducting a more thorough decluttering process at the start of each new season. This is a great time to reassess your belongings, rotate seasonal clothing and decor, and let go of items that no longer serve you.

6. Mindful shopping habits: Develop mindful shopping habits that align

with your minimalist values. Before making a purchase, ask yourself whether the item is truly necessary, whether it aligns with your personal style and values, and whether it will add value to your life in the long term. By being intentional about what you bring into your home, you can prevent clutter from accumulating in the first place.

By establishing routines and habits that support your minimalist lifestyle, you can create a sense of structure and consistency that makes maintaining your minimalist home feel like second nature. Remember, it takes time to develop new habits, so be patient with yourself and celebrate the small wins along the way.

One-In-One-Out Rule

The one-in-one-out rule is a simple but powerful strategy for maintaining a clutter-free home over time. The basic premise is this: for every new item that comes into your home, one item of equal or greater value must go out. This helps ensure that the overall volume of your possessions remains stable and prevents clutter from slowly creeping back in.

Here are some tips for implementing the one-in-one-out rule in your minimalist home:

1. Define your categories: Determine the categories of items that you'll apply the one-in-one-out rule to. This might include clothing, books, kitchen gadgets, or any other area where you tend to accumulate excess items over time. By being specific about which categories you're targeting, you can be more intentional and focused in your decluttering efforts.

2. Be mindful of new purchases: Before bringing a new item into your home, consider whether it truly adds value to your life and whether you're willing to let go of something else in exchange. This mindfulness can help curb impulse purchases and ensure that you're only bringing in items that

genuinely enhance your life.

3. Choose items of equal or greater value: When selecting an item to remove in exchange for a new one, choose something of equal or greater value. This doesn't necessarily mean monetary value, but rather the item's usefulness, relevance, or importance to you. By letting go of items that no longer serve you, you create space for new items that better align with your current needs and values.

4. Be proactive about decluttering: Rather than waiting until you bring a new item home to declutter, be proactive about identifying items that you no longer need or want. Keep a donation box or bag in a convenient location and add items to it as you come across them in your daily life. This ongoing decluttering process makes it easier to find items to remove when you do bring something new into your home.

5. Make exceptions for essential items: There may be certain essential items that you need to replace or upgrade over time, such as worn-out shoes or broken appliances. In these cases, it's okay to make exceptions to the one-in-one-out rule. The goal is not to create a sense of deprivation or to force yourself to make do with items that no longer serve their intended purpose, but rather to be intentional about what you bring into your home.

6. Involve family members: If you share your home with others, involve them in the one-in-one-out process. Encourage family members to adopt the same mindset and to be proactive about decluttering their own belongings. By making it a team effort, you can create a sense of shared responsibility and accountability for maintaining a clutter-free home.

By implementing the one-in-one-out rule, you can create a sense of balance and equilibrium in your minimalist home. This strategy helps you be more intentional about what you bring into your space and encourages you to regularly reassess the value and relevance of your belongings over time.

Regular Decluttering and Reassessment

Even with the best intentions and habits in place, it's natural for clutter to accumulate over time. That's why regular decluttering sessions and periodic reassessments of your belongings are essential for maintaining a minimalist home.

Here are some strategies for incorporating decluttering and reassessment into your minimalist lifestyle:

1.  Schedule regular decluttering sessions:  Set aside dedicated time for decluttering on a regular basis.  This might be a few hours each month, a full day each quarter, or whatever frequency works best for your lifestyle and needs.  By scheduling these sessions in advance and treating them as non-negotiable appointments, you're more likely to follow through and make decluttering a consistent part of your routine.

2. Focus on one area at a time: When decluttering, focus on one specific area or category at a time rather than trying to tackle your entire home at once. This helps make the process feel more manageable and allows you to give each item the attention and consideration it deserves. You might choose to declutter your closet one month, your kitchen the next, and so on.

3. Ask key questions: As you go through your belongings, ask yourself key questions to help determine what to keep and what to let go. These might include:
   - When was the last time I used or wore this item?
   - Does this item bring me joy or add value to my life?
   - If I didn't already own this item, would I buy it again today?
   - Does this item align with my current needs, lifestyle, and values?

By being honest with yourself and evaluating each item critically, you can make more intentional decisions about what to keep and what to remove.

4. Let go of guilt and sentimentality: One of the biggest barriers to decluttering can be feelings of guilt or sentimentality around certain items. You might feel guilty about letting go of a gift from a loved one, or struggle to part with items that hold sentimental value, even if you no longer use or need them. Remember that your memories and experiences are not tied to physical objects, and that letting go of an item does not diminish its significance or the love and thought behind it.

5. Reassess your storage solutions: As you declutter and reassess your belongings, take a critical look at your storage solutions as well. Are your current systems working effectively, or do they need to be adjusted or upgraded? Look for opportunities to streamline your storage and make it easier to access and maintain your belongings over time.

6. Celebrate your progress: Decluttering and reassessing your belongings can be a challenging and emotional process. Be sure to celebrate your progress along the way and acknowledge the hard work you're putting in to maintain your minimalist home. Take before-and-after photos to visualize the transformation, or treat yourself to a special experience or reward after a particularly successful decluttering session.

By incorporating regular decluttering and reassessment into your minimalist lifestyle, you can ensure that your home remains a reflection of your current needs, values, and priorities. Remember, minimalism is an ongoing journey, not a one-time destination. By embracing the process and committing to regular maintenance, you can create a home that continues to inspire and support you for years to come.

Maintaining a minimalist home requires ongoing effort and commitment, but the rewards are well worth it. By establishing routines and habits that support your minimalist lifestyle, implementing the one-in-one-out rule for managing new possessions, and conducting regular decluttering sessions and reassessments, you can create a living space that remains clutter-free, intentional, and inspiring over the long term.

Remember, perfection is not the goal – progress and consistency are what matter most. Be patient with yourself and celebrate the small victories along the way. With time and practice, maintaining your minimalist home will become second nature, and the benefits of living with less will continue to enrich and simplify your life.

# Enjoying the Benefits of a Minimalist Home

Living in a minimalist home offers a wide range of benefits that extend far beyond the aesthetic appeal of a clutter-free space. From increased time, money, and freedom to reduced stress and improved well-being, the positive impacts of minimalism can transform nearly every aspect of your life.

In this section, we'll explore some of the most significant benefits of maintaining a minimalist home. We'll discuss how living with less can free up more time, money, and mental bandwidth for the things that truly matter, how a clutter-free environment can reduce stress and promote a greater sense of calm and well-being, and how minimalism can help shift your focus from material possessions to experiences and relationships. By understanding and embracing these benefits, you'll be even more motivated to sustain your minimalist lifestyle over the long term.

More Time, Money, and Freedom

One of the most powerful benefits of living in a minimalist home is the increased sense of time, money, and freedom that comes with owning fewer possessions. When you're not constantly managing, cleaning, and organizing an excess of stuff, you free up valuable resources that can be redirected toward the things that truly enrich your life.

Here are some ways that minimalism can lead to more time, money, and freedom:

1. Reduced cleaning and maintenance: The fewer items you own, the less time you'll need to spend cleaning, dusting, and maintaining them. With a minimalist home, you can streamline your cleaning routine and enjoy a tidy space with minimal effort. This frees up time for hobbies, relaxation, and spending time with loved ones.

2. Easier organization and decluttering: When you own fewer possessions, it's much easier to keep them organized and clutter-free. You'll spend less time searching for misplaced items, sorting through overcrowded drawers and closets, and making decisions about what to keep and what to let go. This increased efficiency can lead to a greater sense of control and peace of mind.

3. Lower household expenses: Living with less often means spending less on things like home goods, decor, and storage solutions. You may also find that you're less tempted to make impulse purchases or buy items you don't truly need, leading to increased savings over time. This extra money can be redirected toward experiences, travel, or other financial goals that align with your values and priorities.

4. Increased flexibility and adaptability: When you're not weighed down by an excess of possessions, it's much easier to adapt to changing circumstances or pursue new opportunities. Whether you're looking to downsize, relocate, or simply rearrange your living space, a minimalist home allows for greater flexibility and freedom of movement.

5. More time for self-care and personal growth: By freeing up time and mental energy that would otherwise be spent on managing your possessions, minimalism creates space for self-care and personal growth. You may find that you have more time to pursue hobbies, learn new skills, or simply relax and recharge. This increased focus on self-care can lead to greater overall

happiness and fulfillment.

6. Reduced environmental impact: Owning fewer possessions and being more intentional about your consumption habits can significantly reduce your environmental footprint. By buying less, consuming less, and generating less waste, you can feel good about the positive impact you're having on the planet and future generations.

By embracing the time, money, and freedom that come with minimalist living, you can create a life that is more intentional, fulfilling, and in alignment with your deepest values and priorities. While the specific benefits may vary from person to person, the overall impact of minimalism is a greater sense of lightness, flexibility, and purposeful living.

Reduced Stress and Improved Well-Being

In addition to the practical benefits of increased time, money, and freedom, living in a minimalist home can also have a profound impact on your mental and emotional well-being. A clutter-free environment has been shown to reduce stress, improve focus and concentration, and promote a greater sense of calm and tranquility.

Here are some ways that minimalism can lead to reduced stress and improved well-being:

1. Decreased visual clutter: A minimalist home, with its clean lines, open spaces, and lack of visual clutter, can have a calming effect on the mind. When your environment is free from distractions and unnecessary stimuli, it's easier to relax, focus, and be present in the moment. This decreased visual clutter can lead to a greater sense of peace and tranquility.

2. Improved sleep quality: A clutter-free bedroom, with a simple, comfortable bed and minimal decor, can promote better sleep quality. When your sleeping

space is free from distractions and excess stimuli, it's easier to relax and drift off into a restful slumber. This improved sleep quality can have a positive impact on your overall health and well-being.

3. Increased sense of control: When your home is cluttered and disorganized, it can lead to a sense of overwhelm and lack of control. By contrast, a minimalist home, with its intentional organization and lack of excess, can promote a greater sense of control and mastery over your environment. This increased sense of control can reduce stress and improve overall well-being.

4. Reduced decision fatigue: The fewer possessions you own, the fewer decisions you need to make on a daily basis. When you're not constantly deciding what to wear, what to use, or where to store things, you free up mental energy for more important tasks and decisions. This reduced decision fatigue can lead to increased focus, productivity, and overall well-being.

5. Greater sense of gratitude and contentment: Living with less can help shift your focus from what you lack to what you already have. When you're not constantly striving for more or comparing yourself to others, it's easier to cultivate a sense of gratitude and contentment with your current circumstances. This shift in mindset can lead to increased happiness and overall life satisfaction.

6. Improved air quality: A minimalist home, with fewer surfaces to collect dust and fewer items to harbor allergens, can lead to improved indoor air quality. This can be especially beneficial for those with allergies, asthma, or other respiratory issues. Improved air quality can lead to better overall health and well-being.

7. Increased mindfulness and presence: When your home is free from clutter and distractions, it's easier to be fully present and engaged in the moment. Whether you're enjoying a meal with loved ones, reading a book, or simply relaxing on the couch, a minimalist environment can promote increased

mindfulness and a greater appreciation for the simple pleasures in life.

By reducing stress and promoting improved well-being, minimalism can have a trans formative impact on your overall quality of life. When your home is a source of calm, comfort, and inspiration, it becomes a sanctuary from the chaos and demands of the outside world – a place where you can truly relax, recharge, and be your best self.

Focusing on Experiences and Relationships

Perhaps one of the most significant benefits of living in a minimalist home is the way it can shift your focus from material possessions to experiences and relationships. When you're not constantly striving to acquire more stuff or keep up with the latest trends, you free up time, money, and energy for the things that truly matter – the people and experiences that bring you joy, meaning, and fulfillment.

Here are some ways that minimalism can help you focus on experiences and relationships:

1. More time for loved ones: When you're not spending all your free time managing and maintaining your possessions, you have more time to devote to the people you care about. Whether it's enjoying a leisurely meal together, going for a walk in the park, or simply sitting and chatting, a minimalist lifestyle creates space for deeper, more meaningful connections with loved ones.

2. Increased budget for experiences: By spending less on material possessions, you free up financial resources for experiences and adventures. Whether it's traveling to a new destination, taking a cooking class, or attending a concert or sporting event, a minimalist budget allows for more experiential spending that creates lasting memories and enriches your life.

3. Shift in values and priorities: Living with less can help clarify your values and priorities, shifting your focus from external validation and material success to internal fulfillment and meaningful experiences. When you're not constantly comparing yourself to others or striving to keep up with societal expectations, you're free to pursue the things that truly light you up and bring you joy.

4. Increased presence and engagement: When you're not distracted by clutter or the constant pursuit of more, it's easier to be fully present and engaged in the moment. Whether you're enjoying a conversation with a friend, savoring a delicious meal, or exploring a new place, a minimalist mindset allows you to fully immerse yourself in the experience and appreciate the richness of life.

5. Deeper sense of connection and community: By focusing on experiences and relationships rather than material possessions, minimalism can foster a deeper sense of connection and community. When you're not competing with others or trying to keep up with the Joneses, it's easier to build authentic, supportive relationships based on shared values and interests.

6. Greater appreciation for simple pleasures: Living with less can help you rediscover the joy and beauty in life's simple pleasures – a warm cup of coffee, a beautiful sunset, a heartfelt conversation with a loved one. When you're not constantly seeking the next big thing or the latest gadget, you develop a greater appreciation for the small, everyday moments that make life meaningful.

7. Increased generosity and giving: When you're not consumed by the pursuit of material possessions, you may find that you have more resources – both time and money – to devote to causes and organizations that matter to you. Whether it's volunteering at a local charity, donating to a favorite non-profit, or simply being more available to help friends and family in need, minimalism can foster a greater sense of generosity and giving.

By shifting your focus from material possessions to experiences and relationships, minimalism can help you create a life that is rich in meaning, connection, and purpose. When you prioritize the things that truly matter – the people, places, and experiences that bring you joy and fulfillment – you create a life that is not only simpler and more intentional but also more deeply satisfying and rewarding.

Living in a minimalist home offers a wide range of benefits that can transform nearly every aspect of your life. From increased time, money, and freedom to reduced stress and improved well-being, the positive impacts of minimalism are far-reaching and profound.

By owning fewer possessions and being more intentional about your consumption habits, you free up valuable resources that can be redirected toward the things that truly enrich your life – hobbies, self-care, personal growth, and meaningful experiences with loved ones. A clutter-free environment can also promote a greater sense of calm, focus, and overall well-being, creating a sanctuary from the chaos and demands of the outside world.

Perhaps most importantly, minimalism can help shift your focus from material possessions to experiences and relationships – the things that bring true joy, meaning, and fulfillment to life. When you prioritize the people and experiences that matter most, you create a life that is not only simpler and more intentional but also more deeply satisfying and rewarding.

As you continue on your minimalist journey, remember to celebrate and savor the many benefits of living with less. Embrace the increased time, money, and freedom that come with a clutter-free home, and allow yourself to fully enjoy the peace, clarity, and contentment that minimalism can bring. By staying focused on your values and priorities and letting go of the excess that no longer serves you, you'll create a life that is rich in meaning, purpose, and joy – a life that truly reflects your authentic self and your deepest desires.

# Conclusion

Throughout this book, we've explored the trans formative power of minimalism and its potential to create a home and life that are more intentional, meaningful, and fulfilling. From the initial spark of inspiration to the practical strategies for decluttering, organizing, and maintaining a minimalist space, we've covered a wide range of topics and ideas designed to help you embrace a simpler, more purposeful way of living.

As we come to the end of this journey, it's important to remember that minimalism is not a destination but rather an ongoing process of growth, discovery, and self-reflection. It's a way of life that challenges us to question our assumptions, let go of what no longer serves us, and focus on the things that truly matter – our relationships, our experiences, our personal growth, and our overall well-being.

Embracing Minimalism as a Trans formative Journey

Embracing minimalism is not just about decluttering your physical space or adopting a certain aesthetic – it's about embarking on a trans formative journey that has the power to reshape every aspect of your life. When you choose to live with less, you're not just creating a more organized and visually appealing home; you're also making a conscious decision to prioritize your values, your passions, and your authentic self.

This journey may not always be easy, and there will likely be challenges and obstacles along the way. You may struggle with letting go of sentimental items, face resistance from family members, or experience moments of doubt or frustration. But these challenges are all part of the growth process – they are opportunities to dig deeper, to question your assumptions, and to reaffirm your commitment to a life of intention and purpose.

As you continue on your minimalist journey, remember to be patient and compassionate with yourself. Embrace the ups and downs, the successes and the setbacks, and trust that each step is bringing you closer to a life that is more aligned with your deepest values and desires. Celebrate the small victories along the way – the decluttered drawer, the donation pile, the newfound sense of clarity and focus – and use them as fuel to keep moving forward.

Most importantly, remember that minimalism is not about deprivation or sacrifice – it's about creating space for what truly matters. It's about letting go of the excess, the distractions, and the noise so that you can focus on the people, experiences, and pursuits that bring you joy, meaning, and fulfillment. It's about creating a life that is rich in purpose, connection, and growth – a life that allows you to be your best self and to make a positive impact on the world around you.

Encouraging Readers to Start Their Own Minimalist Home Transformation

If you've made it to the end of this book, congratulations! You've taken a significant step toward creating a more minimalist, intentional, and fulfilling life. Whether you're just starting out on your minimalist journey or you've been embracing this lifestyle for some time, the ideas and strategies in this book can help you deepen your practice and create a home that truly reflects your values and priorities.

But reading about minimalism is just the beginning – the real transformation happens when you start putting these ideas into action. So if you're feeling inspired and motivated to start your own minimalist home transformation, here are a few tips to get you started:

1. Start small: Remember, minimalism is a journey, not a destination. Don't try to overhaul your entire home and life overnight – start with small, manageable steps and build momentum over time. Choose one room, one category of items, or one habit to focus on at a time, and celebrate your progress along the way.

2. Set clear intentions: Before you start decluttering or making changes to your space, take some time to reflect on your values, priorities, and goals. What do you want to create more space for in your life? What kind of home environment do you want to cultivate? Setting clear intentions can help guide your decisions and keep you motivated when things get challenging.

3. Enlist support: Embarking on a minimalist journey can be easier and more enjoyable with the support of others. Consider enlisting a friend or family member to join you in your efforts, or connect with like-minded individuals through online communities or local meetups. Having a sense of accountability and camaraderie can make all the difference in staying committed to your goals.

4. Embrace imperfection: Minimalism is not about achieving a perfect, Instagram-worthy home – it's about creating a space that works for you and supports your unique lifestyle and needs. Embrace the imperfections, the quirks, and the personal touches that make your home feel like a true reflection of who you are.

5. Keep learning and growing: Your minimalist journey doesn't end when you finish decluttering your home – it's an ongoing process of learning, experimentation, and growth. Continue to seek out new ideas and inspiration, try out different strategies and approaches, and stay open to the possibilities that minimalism can bring to your life.

Remember, your minimalist home transformation is not about achieving a certain look or adhering to a strict set of rules – it's about creating a space and a life that feels authentic, intentional, and deeply fulfilling to you. Trust your instincts, stay true to your values, and don't be afraid to let go of what no longer serves you. With each step you take, you'll be moving closer to a home and a life that truly reflects your best self.

As we come to the end of this book, I want to thank you for joining me on this journey and for opening yourself up to the trans formative power of minimalism. Whether you're just starting out or you've been embracing this lifestyle for some time, know that you have the power to create a home and a life that are rich in meaning, purpose, and joy.

So take a deep breath, trust in the journey, and let your minimalist home transformation be a catalyst for positive change in all areas of your life. Here's to a simpler, more intentional, and more fulfilling way of living – may it bring you all the peace, clarity, and happiness you deserve.

www.ingramcontent.com/pod-product-compliance
Lightning Source LLC
Chambersburg PA
CBHW050822250726

48653CB00006B/2375